Sally 07799863911

Diary of

CW00969789

Diary of an Unborn Child

An Unborn Baby Speaks to its Mother

Manuel David Coudris

Translated by Pat Campbell & Palden Jenkins

GATEWAY BOOKS, BATH

First published in English in 1992
by GATEWAY BOOKS
The Hollies, Wellow,
Bath, BA2 8QJ

© Gateway Books, 1992

First German publication 1985
as Ich Kann Sprechen
by Goldmann Verlag
Translated by Pat Campbell
& Palden Jenkins

Set in 10½ on 12½pt Bembo and Optima, by
Ann Buchan (Typesetters), Middlesex,
Printed and bound by
Billings of Worcester

Cover painting by Alois Hanslian

British Library Cataloguing in Publication Data
A catalogue record for this book
is available from the British Library

ISBN 0.946551.80.4

Contents

Editor's note

Unfortunately some of the wealth of terms available in German is inevitably lost in translation. In editing, in cases where there has been a choice between accuracy-to-the-letter and readability, I have chosen the latter course, seeking to remain true to the bottom-line meaning of what I understand the baby is conveying.

I myself have been involved in midwifery, and in campaigning for more spiritually oriented birth — my first child was born unnecessarily in hospital, the second was at home, and the third was on a community farm in the bath! I can verify that many of the things the baby Manuji mentions within these covers seem to me to be perfectly valid — in fact, exceptionally important.

But it might be that you find the talk of previous lives a bit difficult. Our current civilisation rests on the basis that we have but one life, and it anxiously guards that notion. I personally find it of secondary importance whether or not we have many lives — the issue for me is that, deep within us, we have piles of (mainly unconscious) memories, personal and archetypal memories, often clothed in the garb of other cultures and times — and at various times of life these memories show themselves to us in real-life situations or *gestalts*, or in dreams, or during therapy, or simply while we're lying in the bath doing nothing!

Whether these come from past lives, DNA coding, the collective unconscious or whatever, it is what they do to us which matters: if understanding and fulfilment are our aims, it pays to give awareness to these arenas. As with past lives, modern folk regard channellings such as this as spurious or invalid — meanwhile, the same people implicitly support the proliferation of a world of dangers and contradictions — rationally, of course. Whatever belief system we support, temporary suspension of judgement on issues such as past lives and channelling will reveal a wealth of value and insight in this book, the core of which is human, and drawn from direct experience.

Regardless of our philosophical inclinations, the material here contains rich gems for many people — parents, parents-to-be, midwives, nurses and doctors, psychotherapists, people on a growth path, and anyone interested in a deeper understanding of the human condition.

Please note that, at times, the script requires reading with a here-and-now attitude: this baby is not speaking with the usual explanatory logic or coherent trains of thought that an adult might use, and frequently there are switches of theme or mood which require rapid adjustment on the reader's part.

There is a lot of love and sensitivity in this book, and the parents of Manuji have been brave to expose their personal lives — they demonstrate in this some of the many difficulties which can befall any two good people when they enter into the magnified process of childbirth. It is with the deep wish to help others that Manuji, Mira and René Coudris have written this book, and it is with equal love and care that we have published it. Please enjoy, and find great value!

Palden Jenkins
Gateway Books, 1992.

Preface to the English edition

Seven years have passed since the first printing of the original German version of this book. Readers have sent us around a thousand letters — from pregnant women, fathers-to-be, grandparents and therapists — sharing their thoughts, feelings and (often dramatic) experiences. Today our son's messages are translated into half a dozen languages, and we are glad to see them come out in English. We have added a new epilogue, which we have put in the newly-released fifth German edition, to inform a bit about what has happened since. We hope that Manuji's pioneering activities will bring good to more unborn babies and parents-to-be, offering a new dimension to parenthood. This is our deepest wish.

René and Mirabelle Coudris, Attersee, Austria, November 1991.

Lovingly dedicated to all children of the new time.
They are the hope of our society.

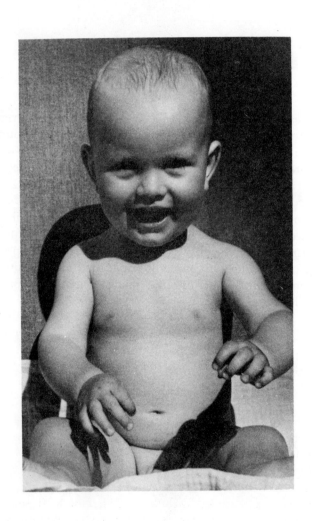

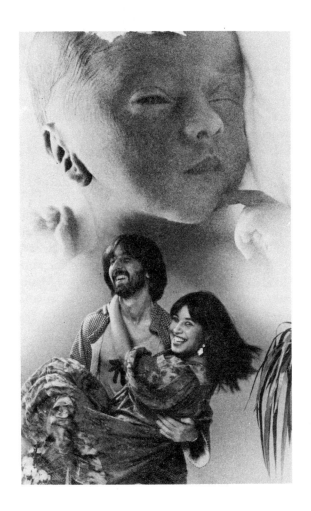

Dear Reader!

In this book the three of us — a baby-to-be and its parents — tell a story about what we have gone through together. It is, in a true sense, a story written by Life itself.

It began on 25th February 1984. On the evening of that day our embryo-baby spoke to us for the first time. Its mother, Mira, more than five months pregnant, was meditating at the time. It announced itself through Mira's inner voice, and the transcripts were simultaneously written down by Mira. We received this with wonder rather than surprise — it was indeed our dearest wish to get into a more direct contact with the baby — but when our wish was granted, we were amazed. We were amazed also with the profound content of the messages, which Manuel David, alias Manuji, gave us — and through this book, gives to all mothers and fathers, midwives, doctors and interested people.

This being, wishing to incarnate, explained that it was coming to us for a purpose. He wanted to help people on earth to reach a better understanding of the nature of the world, of life and love. It took some courage on our part to encompass this — and its likely consequences — especially when Manuji gave us more and more details about his experience as an embryo. Our baby went far beyond the bounds of pre-natal experiences known to science and psychology. We received illuminating answers concerning all sorts of matters.

In the following pages you will find a faithful account of 29 communications, which continued for 44 days, transcribed as they were received. As background, we parents have included a description of the milestones which led up to this phenomenon. We have also included several other relevant stories. In one of the later chapters you will find a surprising final message which we received exactly one year after his birth — just before we went to print.

We are fulfilling Manuji's wish to make public his 'monologues from the womb'. This wasn't easy for us as parents, but we nevertheless felt compelled to publish them in book form. We feel that Manuji's message encourages a more child-oriented and humane society. We were therefore willing to reveal part of our private life for the sake of the children of the future.

The fantastic but completely real series of incidents commented on by us here took place in Austria. It might equally well have happened to you too, and it could equally well have happened in any other part of the world. We very much hope that our report will inspire other parents to consider careful experimentation in this. The first step towards it is simply to take seriously the idea that communication with an unborn child is possible — it doesn't start at birth. Every mother should know that she is able to speak with the child in her womb, in her own way, before birth. Fathers too can establish an affectionate relationship with their child. The father's main task is to encourage and support the mother — and thereby the child. With direct communication, the father can play a more involved role in the baby's pre-natal life. Everyone's lives are changed by it, and people can draw strength from such experiences right to the end of their lives.

Contact between Manuji and us did not come out of the blue. It was encouraged by years of commitment to inner growth. Our meditation practice had paved the way for this experience. Our own baby's initiative could be seen as part of a historical transition period in which even the tiniest inhabitants of our planet participate.

We are living in a time of radical transformation, in a turbulent, even chaotic, period of social change. It is also a time of baby boom: according to United Nations figures, more than 100 million babies are born annually. These children of modern times will soon be taking an active part in the influencing the world. We authors feel a connection with this process of worldwide change. Some say that, in the new epoch, the paranormal will again be accepted as the normal, as has happened in previous times. Perhaps our work is a little piece in an evolving jigsaw of consciousness.

The baby's various physical, psychic and spiritual viewpoints often overlap in a subtle way, or imperceptibly merge into one another. Although Manuji sometimes transmits from dual levels of experience (a baby and a wise one), and then again from an undivided viewpoint, it is always the conscious and alert spirit of the little being which is speaking!

We would like to make one request to the reader in Manuji's own words: *"One must feel and know what is behind the words.*

Then understanding will come." In this light, we welcome your involvement and openness, and would be happy to hear from you if you are moved to write (through the publisher).

Attersee, Austria, March 1985. *René, Mira and Manuel Coudris*

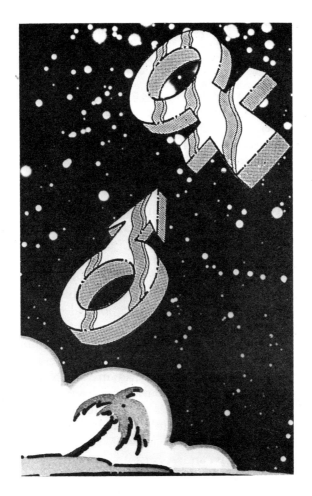

How it all came to pass

René writes . . .

It's difficult, almost impossible, to establish retrospectively when, how and where things began, and to plot their course. Many contributing factors lie far back in the past. Here we give a speeded-up version, a few extracts from and milestones in our past.

It's 1979. We two parents had not yet met. I, René, Manuel's father, was on a protracted journey through Sri Lanka. For months on end I was travelling, enjoying the culture and landscape of that 'happy island', not unmixed with a little shipboard romance. I wanted to settle there and turn my back on the Austrian bureaucratic mentality which had, with a few legal dirty tricks, blocked me from attending a master class at an art university. However, things did not turn out as expected: all that is now left of that trip to Sri Lanka is a few diaries recording my colourful experiences.

Without doubt, the most important occurrence was the 'chance' meeting with a native magician, with whom I did a six-week stint of spiritual practice. He taught me, amongst other things, a Buddhist form of meditation called *Ana-panasati*, by which I succeeded in consciously separating my spirit from my body, seeing the auras of plants and many other things. His clairvoyant faculties were astounding — almost every day he fair blew me away with this. I had my doubts about his pronouncements on my future, but, since then, a great deal (but not everything) has turned out as he predicted.

He entered into himself and told me a lot about a very pretty young woman with long black hair — this filled several pages of my diary. He even gave me an exact description of a birthmark on my future wife's body. He fixed the time when I should meet her at 'two to two-and-a-half years hence'.

After two and a half years, I had given up looking for a fulfilling relationship. I had taken employment in my brother's natural food shop in Vienna, in order to rescue my finances. In the shop, my younger brother's girlfriend was sitting drinking tea with a young woman with short hair, dressed in a very unbecoming manner. Shortly before I came in, my brother's girlfriend had mentioned me. I started talking with this woman, and we landed up together at the cinema that evening. We were suddenly getting close.

Right at the beginning of the film, Rajah guru's mysterious prediction came into my mind. This lady, snuggling up to me, had very dark hair — but it wasn't long. "*I had it cut a fortnight ago, in a fit of self-punishment*" was her passing remark. A few days later Mira left her post in the kindergarten, where she had already given notice months before, and drove with me the 200km (125 miles) back to Linz, to my lodgings. Since those unforgettable days we have been living together and are — in the deepest sense — one heart and one soul. Two years later, on my thirty-third birthday, we got married.

One other curious development arose out of my search for a meaningful partner. After reading an article, I sent off for information from a British professor who had succeeded in dreaming consciously at night. During a period of three weeks' seclusion, I was successful in obtaining a special dream. For one or two seconds I saw the smiling image of a dark-haired beauty who corresponded more or less to Rajah's description. At once a sense of inner certainty that 'she' was the one and that she really existed came to me. Two years later, the same visual situation arose as I had had in that dream.

Of course I went on with my conscious dreaming. The greatest difficulty I encountered, apart from that of maintaining waking consciousness during sleep, was the finding of the right bed. I needed a 'bed of clouds', on which the dreamer's body can lie properly for dreaming. Since I could not find the right bed in the shops, I laboriously constructed on by hand. All my friends saw this and wanted one too, and I recognised a gap in the market. For two years, together with my dream wife, who had turned up by then, I produced these fleecy woollen mats — Japanese-style futons. Later, we sold the know-how about our product under licence to a friend's firm.

We staged four week-long seminars for two directors of a French spiritual centre at the Salzkammergut. I acted as coordinator, Mira did the wholefood cookery (nutrition was one of our shared interests) and over a hundred people came. However, in our enthusiasm we had miscalculated, and it all ended in

financial catastrophe. Nevertheless, we gained many new experiences — in one, we found an enhanced spiritual understanding
of the world, and in the other, Mira's outstanding sensitivity
crystallised and clarified. About this, it's best she tells you
herself.

Mira writes . . .

At about the same time as René was discovering about 'me' in
Sri Lanka, a new phase of my psychic and spiritual development
had begun. I was beginning to take my life into my hands. I had
started with this eight years before, when, at 19, I had, on
impulse, radically changed my attitude toward myself and my
life, and with it my diet. All my troubles suddenly took on a
new light, for within me, a tender seed of new consciousness
was beginning to grow. It's generally known as mediumship.

As far back as I can remember, extrasensory perception
wasn't *extrasensory* for me — it was normal. When I was a little
girl, my grandmother would tell me about her 'super-sensory'
experiences, and for my mother too, such feelings are familiar.
Yet these deep impressions are neither extra- nor super-sensory,
but inward-sensory! Our 'sixth sense' is actually one which acts
as a mirror-image to the outward-oriented senses. I venture to
assert this because since my childhood I have been in more or
less conscious communication with elementals and higher
beings, invisible to the physical eye. More than once I have been
able to grasp the helping hand of these radiant friends, and each
time these penetrating experiences have affected me fundamentally.

I've been inclined to be cautious and shy in demonstrating
these things. I am convinced that such phenomena can neither
be fully reported nor scientifically proven to a satisfactory
degree. Either one has the experience and knows, or else one
does not. Inner knowledge of it is all that counts. The truth is
that almost everyone has these experiences almost all the time,
without realising it. It begins when you feel sympathy or

antipathy for someone. Can you see what it is that causes such feelings to arise within you?

I work on the basis that I brought my intuitive tendency with me into the world. Several earlier episodes confirm this. At three years old I began collecting herbs in the fields. Even at that age I wanted to make them into a healthy soup. I picked all the green plants I could find, except grasses. I brought the greens into our kitchen and demanded a cooking pot and a wooden spoon. My mother put a stool before the stove, so I could reach the hob. I was as happy as a queen with my concoction, and with the strong smell it was giving out. In my opinion, such a witch-like image cannot arise from this life, since I had never heard of such culinary activities in my parents' house. Another experience I had at an early age was floating, or levitating. It only happened once, and it *happened*, rather than my doing it. My parents weren't in the room. A sort of breath of air lifted me up, and gravity had gone. I found myself horizontal, at a height of about half a metre, all lightness and joy. It lasted for perhaps a few minutes, although I had no sense of time. Today, whenever I remember it, a strange feeling of freedom comes over me.

All these talents of early childhood soon faded away. School and the normal social processes did their usual damage. It became more and more seldom that a hint of my suppressed sensitivity would penetrate the veil. Almost 25 years were to pass before this 'paranormal gift' (which I am sure hides within each of us) came properly to the surface again.

During my puberty, only a few glimpses of inner light came through. Otherwise, most of my childhood experiences are more like a nightmare. It was really my intention to become a kindergarten teacher, but my mother's gentle persuasion made me go to the polytechnic college for professional women. At that time I was already up to my neck in psychic problems. I often felt myself driven close to a cliff, and, more than once, was on the edge of plunging over the edge. At that time nearly everyone around me was stuck in an emotional bog. My life-situation was also hopeless and bleak. I felt as if I had reached the end of an oppressive life — yet somewhere inside me I was conscious that life was 'only a cage' in which I found myself, though I had no idea where the door to freedom might be.

With this damaged psyche I slid — still a schoolgirl — into my first marriage, with a sports instructor, 12 years older than I and more than a head taller. After knowing him for two years, I had married him, though only because I had become pregnant and wanted to give the child security. I was certainly not mature enough for such a relationship, and neither was he.

At 17, I had visited a gynaecologist in order to have contraception explained to me. The doctor said that I did not need contraception, since my chances of giving birth were exceptionally slim, and the probability of carrying for one full term was practically nil. I was very surprised, since I had been certain I could have children, just because I love them so much. On the other hand, I comforted myself in the thought that I would not have to bother about contraception, since my husband did not want children.

Several times I sought to extricate myself from this relationship, and finally I landed up with my mother again. Through her, I soon joined a sect, whose name I can no longer remember. In their prayer room I had my first real contact with Jesus. I prayed to him to show me the way out of my unhappiness. While praying, I was enveloped in a shining beam of light, and I cried a great deal. That experience brought about a great inner change in me, and for a long time I kept it to myself.

All the same, I had not really managed to detach myself from my first relationship. Erhard simply fetched me back, and very soon afterwards I realised that I had run away pregnant. When I refused to marry him, he boxed my ears. Under pressure, I finally gave in, because I did not want anything to happen to my baby. I was very tearful and hysterical after making this decision. The gynaecologist said it would be very difficult to carry the baby full term, "but let's wait and see". I watched my growing tummy and physical changes. I loved my baby, but no unusual conversations took place between me and this embryo. One night in the fifth month I got bad back pains and cramp. I thought I had wind and went to the loo, but I began to bleed. Suddenly the pains became very bad, and my husband dragged his feet over driving me to the doctor. The doctor wasn't home, so we had to drive to the hospital in Vienna. The entrance to my womb was already wide open, and for three days and nights I hung on with infusions to stop the pain. I told a nurse that the baby was coming, but she wouldn't believe me. Yet my son soon arrived. Just before the birth I could feel him kicking, and I could hear his heartbeat through the monitor. He weighed 700 grams, and was about the size of my hand — he died during birth.

My husband was glad he was dead. I was more inclined to push everything out of my mind — I was simply in a state of physical collapse, and at the end of my tether. Friends said: "The fellow really hates you, can't you see that?" With my last strength I wanted to be divorced, but nothing came of it. He did not take me seriously. At that time I saw a modest little information sheet stuck in the window of a health food shop. It gave the principles of traditional oriental nutrition. This struck a slumbering chord of knowledge in me. I went at once into the shop and bought unpolished rice — and that was the first gentle beginning of a brightening period of life.

I became convinced that there must be a way out of human misery, and decided that persistent searching would reveal something. Since I had stomach and bowel problems it was obvious I should look for the best possible diet. I understood that the right diet could influence my psyche and spirit, but I did not know how to go about having a good diet. I experimented, and then found a seminar on Yin and Yang by a man named Zeané Lao Shin. My husband threw scorn on me. Yet, during the first few minutes of the seminar, indescribable things happened. A radiation proceeded from this little man, like a lightning flash through the dark mist surrounding me. I was enjoying the first steps on my path.

Zeané was a Taoist priest who had been sent to the West by his Asian master to teach here. The most striking thing about him was his agility, lightness and unsentimental love. This enfolded me as if in a golden cloud, in which no harm could possibly come to me. I came to practise the Zen meditation he taught, and studied the deep insights of macrobiotics. My energy began returning. Later, I went on a holiday, and fasted on miso soup (a traditional Japanese fermented soya-bean broth) and tea: this gave me so much vitality that I felt I could dance the whole night through. I was almost afraid of my strength. Also, on this trip, I fell in love. When I got home, I was caught between my rising strength, and a desire to avoid Erhard's crazy reactions. I distanced myself from him once again.

There grew inside me, however, a desire to have a child. Perhaps this would improve our married life. Erhard neither agreed nor disagreed. Three weeks later, I was pregnant, and was very happy about it, despite finding the atmosphere around me oppressive. I found myself talking a lot to the embryo within, in an indefinite way. Probably more mothers than one supposes do this, despite a taboo against such 'foolishness'.

In the fifth month, however, we came to blows over petty domestic matters. Shortly after, I had a dream in which I was bleeding internally, and then I had the baby, whose eyes were closed, who kicked a little and then died. A week later, exactly that happened: I delayed going into hospital to avoid the interventions they make, and suffered overnight, then went to hospital, and delivered twenty minutes later, three months premature. The baby was taken from me at once — I wasn't even allowed to touch him. He lay in an incubator, trying to breathe. I could hardly look, for the experience was so terrible. I whispered the baby's name — David — and he felt it and tried to turn his head toward me. When he couldn't make it, he moved his little toes skilfully. His body had an unearthly beauty. After thirty minutes, I was taken away for treatment. I believe he died just as the door was shut behind me. When I came back, the incubator was empty. That was too much for me, and I was unable to grasp it: I was in shock, unable to feel anything except emptiness. I asked for my husband, and was told he had gone home straight after bringing me to hospital.

Soon after this, my breasts became filled with milk, which dripped down me, and I was becoming feverish. I was given tablets which then gave me heart difficulties. So there I stayed, in a ward full of cancer patients. Added to this, the doctors developed a prejudice against me because I refused the hospital food, and also a blood-transfusion. After three days, I signed a form and went home on my own responsibility. At home, I felt David's spirit, and this comforted me, so I soon managed to deal with the parting, even though I was still deeply shaken.

Six months later, I began to work as a teacher for maladjusted children, and later found the courage to separate from and divorce Erhard. After selling off old belongings, I went with a friend on a round-the-world trip, which ground to a halt in Egypt with dysentery, returned home to Vienna, found that it wasn't 'home', and launched into another phase of psychic torture. Particularly at fullmoons, I felt I was going over the edge: I knew I had to work through my fears, but I didn't know how to go about it. My Japanese teacher had just died, too, so there was no refuge to be found in anyone else.

Nevertheless, I landed up meeting an Australian woman who was a yogi and psychotherapist. She sat down in front of me, and immediately I began to howl. She helped me uncover the violent emotion I had picked up at my father's death. Eventually, she said I needed no more therapy, and that I seemed to be a high-grade medium, intuitive and sensitive. It was my task to make use of these gifts. She recommended Paramahansa Yogananda's book *Autobiography of a Yogi* to me.

Master Zeané had been most important for me, though. He gave me the courage to take on my life-challenges, and also acted as a mirror of my higher self. His death forced me into a greater clarity. This work is carried on by Michio Kushi, who attended a world congress in 1981, which I chose to go to. René also went to this, though we didn't meet amongst the 1000 people there. Independently, we both were impressed by two French teachers, Gérard Bellebon and Solange Guimond — later, we realised that these two had facilitated Manuji's speaking to us, through what they taught.

René writes . . .

The next few years saw a deep involvement growing between us and these two teachers, who ran a centre in Anjou. On their seminars, they would do 'energy transmissions', wherein, after relaxing the participants down, they would enter a trance, and then Solange would go round to each person transmitting energy through her hands. Reactions would vary, depending on each person's openness. "I function only as a channel", Solange would say. They both seemed to have considerable paranormal faculties and knowledge. Gérard once said: "The healing of the human being in his entirety is necessary so that, freed from the yoke of various sufferings, he can come into full possession of his potential. In this way he will taste the fine nectar of his own self and life, and can thereby participate in the transmutation of the world". Gérard also worked with 'Aquarian technology' such as the Mind-Mirror, the Hypnosis-Stroboscope and Form-Wave Generators.

My spontaneous visit to their centre had given me a clear direction in life. In my enthusiasm, I invited these two teachers to visit Austria to give seminars, which Mira and I later organised. Between these seminars, Solange and Gérard have given us some special training: since Mira had emerged as a gifted medium, they helped us to develop a state of conscious deep trance. They taught us techniques, and worked to clear away our psychic blocks — or at least, the most stubborn ones — and Mira progressed quickly. In the two years which followed, we both zealously practised these techniques. In the course of our trance exercises, we made numerous contacts with our unconscious and super-conscious and with beings beyond our own dimension. When it was confirmed that we were to have a baby, Mira stopped our weekly 'readings', because she did not want to unduly influence the baby.

In retrospect, all this, together with the hardships we each and both went through, were necessary preliminaries to what happened with Manuji. We were able to serve as a 'speaking tube' for him, which itself has led to much, much more. It's funny how hardship and receiving inner gifts seem to go together!

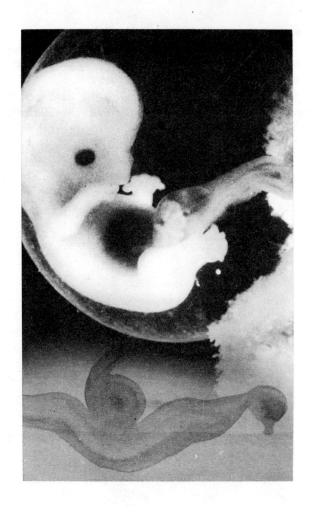

Dreams and visions

Written by Mira

At a young age, I began to take as much interest in my dream world as in my 'real' experiences. I grasped early on that in my nightly looking-glass world I would come upon explanations and perceptions which would enable me to solve any problems. Increasingly I learned to distinguish between unimportant dreams and those which were vital to me. The dream I had about the death of my father remained a puzzle to me for a long time — it was only in adulthood that I came to realise that my unconscious was maturely preparing me for something. Without having read anything about 'dream techniques', I already knew much. For example, if, just before falling asleep, I wished that I could dream about something in particular, this dream would come on that or subsequent nights, either directly or in code. During my puberty, I studied the Bible thoroughly. I could not understand what could be the meaning of the 'Last Judgement'. So I prayed to God to give me an answer, and here is the dream:

"I see myself in wooded countryside with a group of people. We are all lying in hollows and ditches waiting anxiously. Is the Last Judgement coming now? Are we going to see Jesus? Suddenly we all become unconscious. I don't know how much time passes, but I regain consciousness alone. All the others are either dead or gone. My hair has been burnt off and there are great cracks in the ground. Uprooted trees and corpses are lying everywhere. I stand up in amazement, feeling weightless. I feel a finer energy flowing through me. I survey the death and destruction without emotion. I feel as though new-born, and know there is a long way to go before I meet other survivors."

To me, this dream showed the meaning of the second coming of Christ as being permeated with a new, higher form of energy. I can only describe it as feeling totally free. As time went on, the world of dreams became more and more important to me, and so, since then, I have kept records of many of my dreams. In the case of important dreams which I do not understand, I meditate on them until I see their message. I am convinced that with a little patience and help at the beginning, everyone can become his or her own interpreter of dreams.

Dreams can be so useful! The night before I wrote this piece,

I dreamt I was visiting my homoeopathic doctor. On the previous evening I had decided to visit him during the next few days, but in my dream he gave me his advice, and I came to follow it, and a visit became unnecessary! I could give many other examples, but want to mention just a few concerning Manuji. All of these, except that which follows, came to me early in the pregnancy before I had had my first direct contact with Manuji.

> End of 1982: are we going to have a baby? "René is carrying a little basket in which a baby is sitting upright. It has no hair yet, but it has a majestic expression, like that of a king. It looks at people very seriously with its great dark eyes".

I did not attach great importance to this dream, except that it gave me a feeling of certainty that René and I were going to have a child. When? That of course I did not know.

> Sept 83: am I pregnant? "I am walking over the Danube bridge in Linz, wearing a wide, blue frock. I know in my dream that I am pregnant, but am wearing this to conceal it".

This dream confirmed in me a sense that I was indeed pregnant. I went for a pregnancy test a few days later, and there it was, a thick ring in the test-tube, verifying pregnancy. Up to the third month, no one came to find out I was pregnant, except René.

Some weeks later I had a vision of choosing a name. After a few minutes of meditation, I began to sense the presence of a calm, warm, friendly radiation. Shortly afterwards I saw a beautiful youngish woman arising in my mind's eye. She had noticeable hair, gentle eyes and a long brownish gown. She looked deep into my eyes and said: "You will bear a son and call his name Emanuel . . . ". She said other things too. There was an extra deep peace within me when, fresh and energised, I ended that session of stilling my thoughts.

"Emanuel. What an old-fashioned name" was my first

thought. "We could call him Manu for short". I liked that better. I told René about it. All he said was: "Write it down, write everything down". Later he discovered *Emanuel* to be latinised Hebrew, meaning 'God is with us' or 'God helping us', and *Manu* to be Sanskrit (ancient classical Indian), meaning simply a human being. Manu later became *Manu-ji*, adding the Indian suffix denoting respect or endearment, and our baby later used this as his signature in some later messages. He seemed to like it. So now he's known as Manuji or Manuel.

Here's a dream I had in November 1983:

"My tummy is open. I am playing with a boy and a smaller baby girl inside it. My son says 'Mummy, I want to get out' and is just about to jump out. I answer him 'No, you must stay in there for another hour'. They play a little longer in my tummy, and then they simply leap out. They are already so big that we now go for a walk. The boy is a very lively, tough, wiry, self-willed type, and the girl is extremely gentle, delicate and quiet. I am sunburnt, and am wearing a kind of green khaki ranger's garment with boots to match. Then I see that René is with us, and I can feel that all four of us are very happy." [Six years after this dream, our daughter Samantha was born, whose character fits that of the girl in the dream].

Another, from December 1983:

"My baby has just been born. A son. I have a look at him. He has dark, wide-open eyes and he says 'Mama!'. I feel quite clearly that he knows and understands everything. I ask him: 'What was it like inside the womb?'. He answers: 'When it was moonlight, I submitted to the womb. When it was sunlight, I learned things.' 'What did you learn?' 'Astrophysics.' 'From whom did you learn?' 'From a professor.' Suddenly he is not only speaking, but also moving freely. Even though he has only just been born, his behaviour is that of an adult. There are several people there. They are surprised, and cannot help seeing that there is something unusual about the child.

"The child takes no notice of people's reaction. He makes me feel as if he needs nothing from me, neither emotional nor any other kind of protection — except for feeding, but even then he does that of his own accord. He speaks out freely what he knows about this person and that. They are things which no one from outside could know. Everyone denies what the little one is saying.

"As his mother, I am suddenly confronted with a problem: whom should I believe, my child, or these people? Deep inside, I know Manu is right. But I am unsure about how I should behave — since I often feel I have to justify and defend myself. And Manu doesn't seem to care about my role as mother. He makes me understand that it is not he who is asking something of me, but simply that something is often needed . . .

"At some point he goes to a wall. He points in a certain direction with his hand and indicates to us: 'You should go (or look) there'. No one takes any notice."

Strangely, I phoned my friend Eli about it the next day, and was told that her husband Sylvester had had a similar dream. He had been particularly annoyed by people's ignorant non-reaction. Strangely also, we were soon after invited to visit a professor at an astronomical observatory!

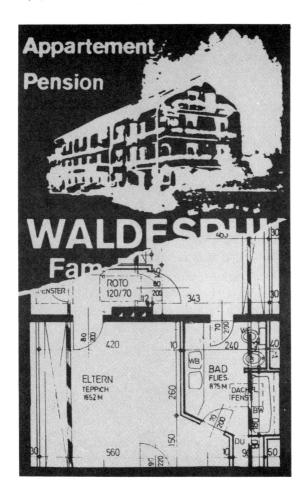

Pregnancy . . . and a better place to stay

Written by René

Both Mira and I grew up in the country, but I was not to remain there for long. My father's career advancement brought us, against my will, to the industrial heart of Austria, and as I grew older, my father's expectations made our family home too small for me. So, from an early age, I stood on my own two feet as regards income and accommodation. This brought me up against the housing market, for here, as elsewhere, rents are so high that many cannot afford to live in proper accommodation. I got used, over the years which followed, to changing my abode often.

Thus, before I met Mira, I was something of a nomad. I also tried many different jobs — technical draughtsman, bookseller, printer, market researcher, commercial artist and student of architecture — and scraped through somehow. I couldn't complain of being bored! But accommodation was my weak spot.

When Mira moved in with me, my lodgings were too small, and the contract was soon ending. Something strange happened there: a tall overloaded bookcase collapsed, falling on Mira. Half an hour later, she miscarried, in about her sixth week. She had been bleeding unusually some days before, but it was only through this accident that we realised that conception had taken place. We then examined the tiny body under a magnifying glass. This re-activated Mira's traumas over motherhood. I mention all this because, in his very first message, Manuji said to Mira: " . . . not much time has passed since I went away from you *unborn*".

Soon after, we moved into an old wooden house built during the war. Here at least we had enough room for our futon-production, our livelihood. The house seemed to be a good deal. A lot of the psychic 'readings' and healings we did happened in one of the rooms there, and Manu mentioned it when talking about his entry into the womb. However, the air in Linz is bad, and in certain unfavourable conditions, Mira could not deal with it — her eyes were often running. She wanted to leave Linz, especially as it emerged that the house was uninsulated and had been declared unsafe for habitation. We looked for somewhere in the country, and no solutions came.

Eventually, though, we found an advertisement for an attic flat in the country, at a place called Pension Waldesruh (Waldesruh meaning 'woodland peace'). That sounded good. On first sight, the place looked like paradise. So we signed a contract to rent the flat. However, later we found we had made a mistake — even Manuji came to comment on our unfavourable quarters.

At first, all was sunshine. We were the first to move into the new block, and the good weather had disguised its draughtiness. Also, we had attached no importance to all the flies lying dead on the floor when we had viewed the flat. Little problems which we thought at first we could fix increased during our first year there, and became really difficult. The house stands on a hill, and, despite attempts to insulate and plug gaps, the draught simply found other ways in. The house had been jerry-built, with faulty insulation, a chimney which blew back — but a charming view of hills and fields. Sometimes, during storms, it looked as though the whole house would take off. The landlord, meanwhile, gave us empty promises about repairing things.

Later, a sheet-metal works opened up nearby, disturbing the peace — we had to wear earplugs when we were meditating! Nevertheless, after our first winter there, Mira did a course of fasting and purification for several weeks, spending several hours every day meditating and in communication with some of her friends in the spirit world. These gave her an intense spiritual training — which was to be important for Manuji, who entered her body a few weeks later. Then Mira went on a therapy holiday in Majorca with a sick woman who was to receive healing and rest with her. The lady's expectations were narrow and myopic, and her powers of self-healing could not be activated properly. It was quite stressful for Mira, who found her peace in the waves of the sea.

One evening, Mira rang me euphorically to say she was absolutely sure she was to have a baby with me. She was almost obsessed with the idea — Manuji explained this obsession a few months later. When Mira returned, we stayed a night in our town lodgings, out of which we were finally moving all our things. Since we had not made love since before her fast, our attraction was strong. We both felt that evening that we had 'scored'. I soon forgot about it, but when we discovered Mira was pregnant and reckoned back, it must have been that night.

Autumn came, and more tenants moved into the country house. It was only now that things got really unpleasant. Owing to the lack of sound insulation, we could hear everything that went on in the flats below — even words spoken in a normal voice. Banging of doors, trumpet music, and the scuffling of slippers nearly drove us mad. So it was that Mira, sensitised by pregnancy, found refuge in the woods nearby whenever she wanted to recover from being at home! Mira used to wrap her stomach in a thick scarf to muffle the noise for the baby. Already we were discussing where else we could move. Troubles piled upon troubles, and eventually we called a lawyer.

However, the last episode of this affair was only just beginning: we were inundated with house-flies! The buzzing mob would fly around the lamps and collide with the light bulbs all evening, and they would fall into our food or land up lying in dozens, dead on our carpet. Since not even our lawyer or the court could believe such a crazy situation, we asked the local policeman to support us as an objective witness. He was flabbergasted.

While I was flat-hunting, Mira could bear it no longer. She was getting very nervy, and went to stay with a friend — she never came back to the flat. It had only been our love for each other which had kept her there for so long. The court ruled that we needed to pay no more rent or heating costs. When I cleared out the flat some months later, the rain was beginning to come in through the roof!

Nevertheless, we take the view that we need some problems in order to give ourselves a chance to grow inwardly: if we were always content, we'd never get anywhere!

Wie ihr merkt
spreche ich eure
Sprache.
Eigentlich ist es
meine Mutter,
die alle Impulse
die sie durch mich
erfährt
in Worte kleidet
und nieder-
schreibt.

Mediumship with Manuji

Written by Mira

I am very serious and rather more cautious than René about
mediumistic phenomena. They present no problem to me
from the spiritual viewpoint, but my experiences on the psychic
plane have taught me to approach such things cautiously. With

growing understanding of myself I have lost much of this fear, but the knowledge that many other people are not open to psychic realities still leads me sometimes to be over-cautious. Even those who are more open say crazy things, such as: "*Who's a better medium?*". "*Who is closer to God?*", "*So-and-so is a black magician*" and other childish things. Spiritual contests such as these make people insensitive to the real energy of love, and they have become lost in dark suspicions and speculations.

If the magical and the super-sensory were not regarded as special or abnormal, people who are sensitive would be able to carry on their work in a freer, more relaxed manner. Constructive criticism and exchange of experiences could take place, which would benefit everyone. I know that many sensitives would like to talk more about their experiences. As it is, many such people stand alone. If anyone reading this feels this way, you are welcome to write to us.

During my pregnancy, I was averse to doing trance mediumship. Two reasons were behind this: first, the more a person has found a way into him- or herself, the more he or she will have natural access to inner realities without trance; and second, a large measure of psychic stability is necessary before one experiments with the subconscious or super-conscious, and it is generally accepted that the psyche is often unstable during pregnancy.

Successful psychic work can take place only through purified inner channels and a relaxed psyche. At the beginning of my inner training I experienced a huge iceberg, a wilderness of unresolved psychic material, dreams and unresolved problems waiting ready to surface. This led to a kind of pressure against the internal floodgates: my greatest fear was that I was not yet ready to open the gates, that I did not yet possess the psychic strength to stand up to the full force of the flood.

This brought up some differences between René as a man and myself as a woman, for since he is more intellectual than I, he had not gone so deeply into the psychic world. For myself, I feel no inherent dangers in mediumistic work, for it is not psychic things but spiritual growth which I am discovering and seeking. Also I tend to work with the things I know, to apply them, while René goes into things because they're new and stimulating. This may be just a woman's way of looking at things! René finally succeeded in moving me with his argument that I possessed my hidden talents in order to develop them creatively.

René writes:

In the second month of Mira's pregnancy, shortly after a gynaecologist had confirmed it for us, I hit upon the idea of establishing contact, through Mira, with the consciousness of the embryo. Why should it not be possible, between developed spirits, to establish connection with this being who was in process of becoming incarnate? Having experienced many strange things in my life, I believed in the 'possibility of the impossible', beyond the bounds of reason, and such contact seemed perfectly plausible.

Mira refused to have anything to do with it. I was obliged to shelve the idea. But it didn't feel right to do so. Things moved on. As Mira stroked her expanding tummy, she spoke a lot to the baby, in her thoughts or out loud, as if she were speaking to an adult — and the baby showed its reactions through its movements and moods. It happened increasingly. However, I did not have the same direct line to the baby as Mira, and it began distressing me. I stroked Mira's tummy too, but somehow, as a man, I stood separate from their closeness. This brought up deep feelings of sadness.

At the beginning of the fifth month, Mira astonished me by saying that she felt a strong urge to 'listen in' to the baby. She felt the baby had something to say to her. I suggested she get herself into a completely calm state, and then speak to the baby. Since conception, we had not been following our usual psychic practices, learnt from a new age centre in France, and suddenly, here was Mira, running around the flat, getting quite excited about a new way of doing psychic work. Two days later, when she could no longer stand the inner pressure, she made the first serious attempt.

After an exercise to obtain initial opening — usually I would help her tune in to her 'source' — I left her alone with relaxing music in our small bedroom, and lay down on the sofa in the next room. What happened next is best related by Mira.

Mira writes:

A few thoughts about meditation. The first prerequisite for direct contact with the embryo is a harmoniously balanced psyche. The best, and in my view only, way to experience this inner peace is meditation, which can take thousands of different forms, and needs to be well-practised. It's good to start with a definite method, and a teacher is essential at the beginning, although this definite method will recede into the background in the course of time. Yet, the finer points of mediumship cannot be achieved solely with the help of books.

I myself prefer to use a yogic sitting position — cross-legged, upright back and a 'mudra' (or gesture of the hands and fingers) pointing outwards. Or I use a Zen form of sitting, kneeling, with the palms of my hands cupped inwards, resting on my lap. After stilling my thoughts for a while, I enter slowly into the trance state. What happens next is indescribable, and each person needs to experience it for themselves.

During that week an urge had come over me to do my meditation with a paper and pen ready. I felt it had something to do with the baby. I resisted for a few days, then took action. I went into meditation, and a strange feeling came up of being weak in the stomach. René left the tape-recorder running, and writing material — a new cloth-bound Chinese notebook. He meditated with me for a while, then went out.

I allowed myself to sink right down. A growing feeling arose to write everything down. I started writing. My hand hurried the ballpoint over the lines. This inward dictation was so quick that I didn't have time to think. One page after another was filled, as though of its own accord. I simply could not stop, the urge was so great. It didn't come from me . . .

Suddenly there was a loud noise in the flat below. I lost contact and remained stuck in the middle of a sentence. I was too amazed by everything to be annoyed by the interruption. Was I to believe what I had written? What was happening? What will my friends think? I called René and showed him the text.

We read it together and then gazed at each other speechless. René was very happy about it, but I was still uncertain. All evening he was puzzling over what the completed last sentence would have been. We took it in turns to stroke the baby in my stomach, lying cuddled together for hours on end, and then fell asleep.

Thereafter, I felt a strong need to get down to this mediumistic (not automatic) writing, and to take down what this inner voice was saying. Often I did indeed try to break in with my intellect, while I was hurriedly writing down the words and sentences, but I never really succeeded. Before the sessions, I didn't have the faintest idea what the messages would be, or what experiences in our everyday life Manuji would mention. It all became more exciting from day to day, and our relationship with the baby became ever closer. Thus we entered upon a six-week adventure.

Once or twice the texts brought me into conflict with my intellect, self-criticism and fear of being condemned by others. It was quite clear from my feelings that the source was male, though I had my doubts when I read the material afterwards. René helped me unsnag myself from this internal debate by encouraging me to 'stay on the ball' and carry on. Also, I was driven by a strong inner urge, a will-force proceeding from the baby which I was unable to oppose.

The text, as it emerged, was phonetic, and often without punctuation or grammatical correctness. We therefore made corrections to make it readable, but scarcely more than a dozen words were added or removed in order to make sense. Otherwise, what follows is a fully authentic and chronological record of the messages.

Slip now into the world of the smallest of human beings, who up to now have been the least well understood. Feel yourself to be in a forgotten realm, to which we all of us, once upon a time, used to belong . . .

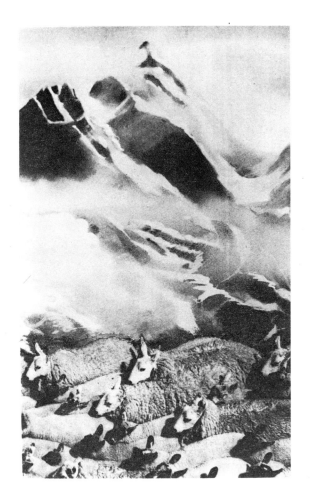

1.   I Come from Far Away

25th week of pregnancy, 1st message.
Pension Waldesruh, February 25th 1984.

I can speak! And you are going to read what I say!
How often it has happened in the past that a being, which was not yet visible, has been able to speak to its friends — the inhabitants of the earth!

Yet my case is rather different.

I am inside the body of a human woman and I have not yet died [from the intermediate state between death and birth], which means for you humans that I have not been born. I come from far away. My spiritual home is the Himalayas. I have been meditating there for many years and preparing myself for this coming.

My mother is a very dear woman, who still has many problems with her psyche and with her 'bodies'. But she has a very great desire to learn. And she knows about going home, about being in inner space, and has it within her power to master this.

Mama, I am David[1], your previous son, but no longer the same one. In terms of earth time, not much time has passed since I went away from you unborn. My mother in this life knows me well. That is why she can love me so much. It is not like that with all mothers.

My story is a solemn, sad and beautiful one. In it I would like to tell you not only what I am but also about my experiences, my adventures, my pasts and, above all, about my present situation. It is a very strange one, since I am one of the first unborn children to be able to take an active part[2].

I thank you for your great openness and your genuine amazement!

It is my desire to help all women understand what is happening when one of us — unseen, unborn and unknown to you — is already living amongst you in the flesh. Until you hear my words, you will not even have suspected how little you people of the earth know about such things.

I am speaking here in the name of many as yet invisible tiny humans. Each of us has endless love. And our understanding is boundless, because with us there is not yet — or rather, there is no longer — such a thing such as *thought*. We *feel* with our whole being, and are totally in the present.

Although we are — as you believe — very much restricted and lacking in freedom living in the little temple of our human mother, we are infinitely freer in our experiences than you can imagine. We have not yet acquired the stamp of your mental imagery and your imagination. We do not yet know hatred, nor do we know fear, but we experience it through our mothers, and what we experience is astonishing.

Now listen! I would like to begin with my previous life on earth, and then I will tell you about my stay in 'heaven', as you call it, and finally, I shall tell you fully about my present life.

It is still some time to my birth, and my mother is allowing me to speak through her. Although mother's circumstances are perhaps rather trying . . . [3]

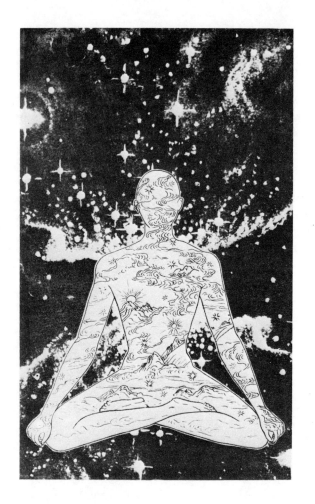

2.   *My Himalayan Life*

25th week of pregnancy, 2nd message.
Pension Waldesruh, February 26th 1984.

. . . she is fiercely determined to go her own way[4].

Mama, I am behind you. Can you feel me? I am embracing
you with my unseen arms and letting my innermost feelings flow

into you, and also all the courage which you now are needing in order to write down everything you receive from me.

You are seeing me now in your mind's eye. And you like me![5]

I am Emanuel. You gave me this beautiful name after a female guardian angel had appeared to you during meditation[6].

As you can feel, I am always accompanied by six spiritual beings, who are there to protect my present life in your womb. It is their task to intercept unforeseen, imbalanced vibrations which might reach me, or to harmonise them by means of their radiant love. One of my spiritual friends also has an inner connection with you. You can contact her at any time[7].

Do not worry about anything any more. All is well. You know how to draw the line under the saying "everything will be alright".

My last life was in and around the Himalayas. I lived as a shepherd, but secretly I had many other interests beside guarding sheep. I lived in a little hut beside a river. There were quite a few goats as well. I grew my own food, and friends often came to see me, and brought me gifts.

A good friend of mine is still living there. He is very, very old — over one hundred years. He makes wonderful music on a pipe he carved himself. His eyes are very pure and shining. How often he helped me, when I was filled with doubt!

I lived alone. All my love and attention was directed toward my spiritual and psychic development. Since early youth I had felt a strong urge toward perfection. I did not have to subject myself to any hard spiritual torture. I never had what you might call frustration, but often I seriously doubted whether I would achieve perfection in that life.

My life was very simple, but the way I led it brought difficulties and complications. In my thoughts I often tried to make a complex, sophisticated life for myself. Yet I was aware I would never lose my inner quietness and simplicity.

I loved my days in solitude by the river, in gentle communication with the trees and other beings. I did not experience any external pressure, but inwardly the desire had arisen to experience something entirely different. Many a time I would let my mind soar to join that of other people living a totally different life, in order to share their experience. I noted how many of them longed for my own lifestyle, since through their inner wishes they had landed in an extremely confused and incomprehensible situation.

When I saw that, I suddenly wanted to experience that very same thing — but with the basis of the calm life inside me. Simply to test what it was like to live in the full bustle of the noisy world — with peace in my heart.

As you see, I speak your language. But actually it is my mother who experiences all the messages from me as impulses, and clothes them in words and writes them down.

There are several ways for us little ones to make contact. One is through the embryo. Everything which goes on in this tiny little body is experienced. But don't think that that is all! My body is swimming around in its 'primordial soup' and is fully occupied with its enormous growth. It is directed solely towards the present moment, its feelings and reactions. I will tell you about this in greater detail.

What you perhaps do not know is that what this body is helping to produce, namely the being of the human-to-come, was always there and always will be! Only, its experience alters its personality — as when after a profound experience you are no longer the same. A similar thing happens to an embryo as happens to you in sleep. It lives without a body, set free, living in the spirit. It is a real experience and it often happens that one wakes up as if from a dream and recognises they both are real — waking and sleeping.

So, I, Emanuel, am speaking to you as an awakened being. My spirit and my little human body are one. My body is developing, to gain the experience I have chosen to have, to help me learn further lessons, and awaken further.

Actually, what's going on here, and what my human-mother is writing down, is as a dream to my little embryo. I — as embryo — experience speaking to you in a dream, yet I am fully conscious (not, I think, in my little body, though I don't really distinguish between my experiences sufficiently to know). Whenever my concentration is directed toward my little body, I forget the dream state — like you when you are awake — in order to go my way totally in the present, without hindrance.

It is good for little babies to 'fall asleep'. On the one hand they must recover from their many experiences and exertions, and on the other they must be free for all the new things they are about to discover.

You will be able to distinguish when I am speaking from my dream-state, and when I am in my little human body.

Perhaps you are beginning to understand why there has as yet been no knowledge about 'before-birth' and 'after-death' amongst the sleeping people of the world.

Do you know that 'before' and 'after' are of the same origin and are, therefore, the same thing? Many people are afraid of death. Why is there so much emphasis on death? Why do so few people ask themselves seriously and boldly "What is birth?".

I tell you, it is one and the same. It is only the stage-play that changes as the curtain rises and falls. You know how it is when you are in the theatre. Before the curtain goes up, no one is unhappy: everyone is full of anticipation. During the play most people forget themselves, and those are the moments they truly long for most! If that does not happen, people get annoyed. They feel cheated out of this self-forgetfulness. They are less concerned with the play itself than with being able to forget their physical bodies by watching the play. After the play there often comes a gentle feeling of wistfulness that it is all over. They must wake up again.

Don't you know that, howsoever things are in childhood, they are also in adulthood?

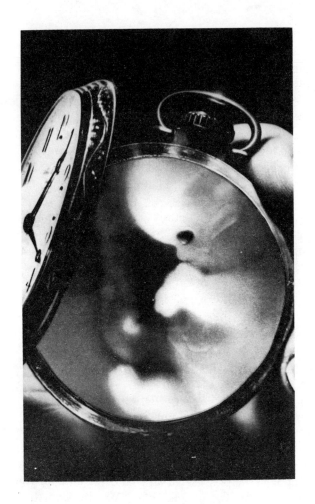

3. Today I Have Experienced a Lot!

26th week of pregnancy, 3rd message.
Pension Waldesruh, February 28th 1984.

Today I have experienced a lot. My mother and father have no
work at the moment, and they have no proper home[8].
Mother is unhappy, because she has not yet found a suitable

place for us to live, and father is annoyed. All the same, they are inwardly in good spirits, without always knowing it themselves.

I am now lying across the womb. My toes are touching the firm, warm flesh of my mother's body which surrounds me. I feel warm and satisfied. The liquid gently enfolds my body. I am firmly tied in the middle with a cord, which sways in the water. I play with it when it touches my fingers. I suck at it too, or touch my face with it.

My ears can already hear very well and my whole body reacts to loud vibrations with jerks or pulling tight. I best like listening to my mother's voice when she is speaking to me. She has been familiar to me right from the very beginning, when I learned to distinguish sounds. Her voice is gentle and comforting. If she shouts, I know she is not speaking to me. When she is speaking to me, her tone is quite different from when she is talking to someone else.

I have also learned to know when she is speaking to my father. That is different again, but the sound gives me a similar feeling to when she is addressing me.

I can recognise my father's voice when he is speaking to my mother — it is quite different from when he is speaking to anyone else. He has not yet spoken to me with his voice, but he has with his hands. I have felt their warmth, and the calm, loving radiation from them. His hands are much bigger than my mother's, and they give me a different feeling.

Whenever my father puts his hands above my womb-dwelling, the feeling which I already have from the warmth of my mother's body also changes. A very faint vibration starts up, as though warmth and light were radiating more strongly. It transmits a total feeling of 'being-safely-hidden-away-with-you'! From the kind of vibration surrounding us, I can feel at any moment whether my parents are preoccupied with me or with something else.

When my mother speaks to me, the rate of my heartbeat rises slightly. I feel my blood circulating more strongly, which brings up in me a feeling of being stretched. My mother's blood also flows more quickly when she sees that I am reacting.

Often, if I have slept longer or if I am just resting inside her, and I want to regain the feeling of being in conscious contact with her, I make stronger movements. Wonderfully for me, my mother lovingly reacts to this immediately. Usually she will speak soothingly to me, or else she will stroke me or give me some other sign, from which I know she is paying attention to me. Some of my mother's body-postures are uncomfortable for me: then I just kick out and my mother immediately knows why and alters her position — usually I immediately calm down.

The best things is when my mother moves her muscles, thus giving me a kind of massage, gentle or hard. This relaxes me — my body goes with the movements. It is as though my mother's hands were in there touching me, stroking and pressing as though to show me that I am there and I am wanted.

The short feeling of tension at the first firm pressure of her muscles makes the blood flow more strongly into certain parts of my body, and then more and more blood comes in waves. It's a kind of tension-relaxation. That is very important for my body, since it is never quite able to stretch out.

The water gives me plenty of freedom of movement. I can move my body without effort. The gentle murmuring, which always remains the same, is a constant accompaniment which soothes me. My mother's heartbeat is always there too, although sometimes the interval alters between the beats.

My mouth was the first opening in my body which I experienced and learned about. What a wonder it is for me! I can reach into the inside of my body with my fingers. That is a deep sensation and gives me 'consciousness-of-myself'.

I can already do quite a lot with my lips. I can distinguish between my individual fingers, and other things. It is great fun to open and shut my mouth, and the waves of the water stroke it pleasantly.

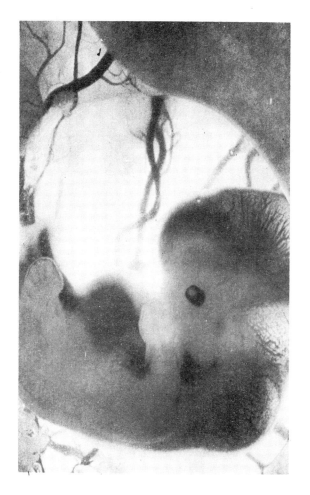

4.   An Embryo Doesn't Think

26th week of pregnancy, 4th message.
Pension Waldesruh, February 29th 1984.

As I have already told you, for an embryo there is neither past nor future. It does not think in the sense that you know. It feels and experiences the real, always in the present.

What it already does do is learn. For example, as you experience a thunderstorm, the little one feels a strong, emotional excitement in its mother. It learns to know what it is like when, not of its own doing, strong waves of excitement from its immediate surroundings not only approach it, but flow right through it.

It learns that every feeling changes, and can distinguish between relaxing, calm feelings, meaning safety, and others which are more heavy, incomprehensible and at times frightening, when they come together. This can cause painful contractions for the little one, though, because it is suddenly left on its own, devoid of any connection with the inner feeling of being at one with its mother.

Such an experience of contractions produces the first feeling of separation for the little one, a feeling of powerlessness, of being forsaken, of 'there is nothing I can do, it just happens to me'.

It may be (and how often this happens!) that the boundless trust, the embryo's relaxed feeling of being totally loved is shaken for the first time in such an instance — unless its mother (as representative of the Great Mother Nature) once again assumes benign control and purposefully establishes full contact with her baby as quickly as possible, making it the focus of her attention, and explaining to it what has happened, physically and mentally. Above all, showing that she, its mother, is there, that she is protecting the baby, and that, in spite of all storms, deep down everything is alright.

Storms are not so bad for a baby — indeed they are actually important — provided that in the course of events it does not become forgotten by its mother. An embryo learns very quickly to have deeper trust if, in a raging storm, it experiences the ongoing loving feelings of its parents.

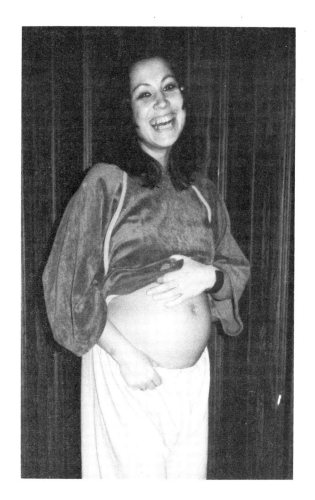

5. Touching Hearts

26th week of pregnancy, 5th message.
Pension Waldesruh, March 2nd 1984.

Yesterday evening I felt that my mother was worrying about me.

At the moment we are living in a house where sound carries

very loudly and every time someone below bangs the door, which happens very often, it is like a physical blow to my mother. I often react a lot to these abrupt vibrations. My mother worries about all this more than I do. I soon recover from the shock of the noise, but sometimes this unpleasant shadow becomes lodged in her mind.

This morning she has regained complete confidence and certainty that we are, in fact, well off.

My Mama! This warm inward beam which now connects us! What immeasurable love and tenderness! You have no words to describe this love! You cannot reproduce our feelings with others. Papa helps us to meet so deeply and warmly as well, with his understanding. All uncertainty disappears when you move inwardly, like that, towards me!

You have seen me! Quite plainly! Before your inner eye![9] You know how I am, what I look like. "It simply cannot be otherwise", you thought to yourself. My wide-open eyes — you have opened them for me now — you are allowing me to be now what I shall be seen to be, months ahead.

Our hearts are touching, my smaller one and your larger one. You know now that my blood is your blood, that our blood and Papa's blood are one. How lovely!

As yet we have not discovered separation — we shall talk about this later. We are a unity, but not a unity in the psyche — not one like most people imagine. Many people act solely in accord with a self-created clinging attachment, rooted in fear and ignorance . . .

But right now, let's give ourselves to this deep music[10]. Waves of music stream through you, relaxing both our bodies completely. Like this, there is no demarcation, as if our bodies didn't exist.

We are both here and we know it. I am holding the umbilical cord in my right hand. My left hand is moving freely. I sense waves of joy.

You know that I am not saying these words. Don't worry —

you are writing the right words for our common impulses. I am speaking inside you.

Is it not so that we, all of us, speak not only in words? What is more, words are often a covering for something quite different. A message must be felt. Behind words one must feel and know. Then there will be understanding.

I like sucking my thumbs. That came quite by itself — like when an idea first comes to you.

I hear the sounds you make. They are always around me, and this continuity gives me security. I feel how happy you and René are with me. When I lie between you and we can feel each other completely, there is no longer any question of being alone or of 'loving only you'.

You know now what it means — from unity — to be born into 'separate unity'.

Everything is symbolic. Our father in 'heaven' also gave birth to us.

Jesus is with us. I can often see him as a beaming light — and you then tell me that one of our best friends is with us.

To me it makes no difference whether you are thinking of someone, whether someone is there in the flesh or appears in a subtle body, invisible to other humans. I sense all who are present. And I can distinguish between them.

You have come to understand the need to choose between your friends. I thank you for that.

My friend, little Daniel, is in his Mama's tummy, as I am. We often exchange vibrations. He is well, and he is already looking forward to his arrival, as is his Mama. He does not communicate with her as we do, but he is just as well as I am, because he is wanted and loved. His mother believes that she must wait for some time longer until she sees him, and before she can speak to him. But his little sister often speaks to him in her dreams. She tells her mother about it.

You received a letter yesterday, and it made you very happy! I would like to give you a poem:

In the deep lake
there is a lotus blooming
forsaken and alone.
Yet those
who only look with outer eyes
just recognise the appearance
and believe they are alone.
Nevertheless,
whoever looks behind this
with tranquillity
becomes filled with delight:
How wide and beautiful, how deep
God's universe blesses us.

I wanted to tell you, I'm often with you in your dreams! Sometimes you do not notice me at all, or see me.

I was restless in the night. Before that I had felt a constriction like cramp above my head. It began after a man had called. He said things which left an impression on you[11]. Since you neither held on to it, nor could you get it out of your head, it brought on a stomach cramp (as you call it). I could feel you trying to relax it, but you weren't successful, because you had allowed yourself to be deeply stirred.

It did not worry me too much, except that I felt fewer energy-sources flowing into my own sphere. You then did an exercise[12] and altered your breathing, and that helped you. We then lay down, and soon you had a severe ache in your chest. Then you let energy flow into the place through your hands — that did me a lot of good too.

I can hear the birds twittering through you and can feel what they are saying. So much joy! Whenever you hear the birds singing, you immediately feel happy. It touches you like a love-filled spell.

The birds in the wood. And the wood itself. When you feel you want to give me more rest, you go with me to the woods. For the moment all is well.

My toes are playing in the water. I can move each one of them very well. The soles of my feet are very sensitive and I often stroke them across the inside of your tummy.

Often you have no idea that a specific feeling which comes over you is really from me. If I stroke very gently across your inside, you still feel it, even in places where you have no nerve-ends.

I try to touch you from inside. And when I turn, you distinctly feel it. Often a warm feeling of joy arises in you when I am feeling very well.

Today I pulled a little at the umbilical cord. You noticed it and turned a little. Then you laughed a lot, differently from your usual laugh. Not outwardly, but inwardly. It came quite of its own accord from deep inside you. You became aware of it and knew it had something to do with me[13].

You have so many questions to ask me![14]

But today I don't want to talk about serious things. Let's call a halt to the writing.

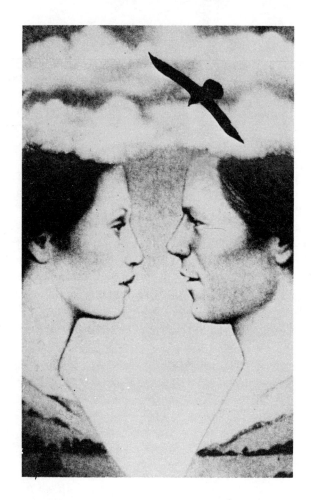

6. *All is Well*

26th week of pregnancy, 6th message.
Pension Waldesruh, March 3rd 1984.

M y Mama! We are growing closer and closer. You cried as
you came down ever deeper to meet me. Now I am quite
still, I am with you. I am living inside you! Like me, at this very

moment [in your meditation] you are experiencing that you are not your body, but that you are simply inhabiting it. And yet both of us are in our bodies.

I am like your subconscious. You can currently see me only if you sink down quite deep in yourself and touch me. You feel me. I feel your caressing and loving waves lapping around me.

My Mama! Yes, I am here!

How many women there are who don't know the unborn baby inside them! It's like their unfulfilled dreams: they do not dare to approach what is inside them, of which they are unconscious, for fear of experiencing something unpleasant. They do not trust themselves to meet the feelings they usually keep in check, and the memories of which they are not conscious. Nevertheless, these feelings and memories live on secretly inside, like mountains of energy locked away.

I am your present, your utterly-present beingness in the subconscious and the superconscious. Why is it that so many people spend their time looking outwards rather than within?

I will speak now about these poor women and children, who, merely from unknowing, are always ill and unhappy. Many women believe in clinging to the past. They do not believe that, overnight, they could do away with so much of their unnecessary psychological ballast. Because of this lack of belief, this release just doesn't happen. Even in their imagination, such people have no feeling that they could let go of all that has already fulfilled itself and come true.

Everything is good just as it is.

If only, through love of their baby, women were able to lose their own fears! If only they could believe in the courage and the power of the new one, instead of throwing all of their own ballast onto what is new and pure. Naturally, such women have children in order to learn from such situations.

I know that you do not believe in the power of your own great divine will. Therefore you first follow the way of the mind. Very slowly, step by laborious step, you chew over all the facts and experiences which have already happened in the past. Looking at these clearly, they should demonstrate the causes of all misfortune — but no, this doesn't happen! For, through your attitudes and beliefs you attract to yourself all the kind of unfortunate events, conditions and factors which you seek to avoid. So there are unlucky people everywhere — it's a matter of, first, believing in freedom.

There is an exercise you can do: imagine yourself being set free. This exercise is successful only for those who have, however, taken the first steps toward freedom.

As we grow, we little ones in the womb begin to experience the suffering which comes when people believe only in their own limited experience, and cannot give anyone their freedom, either in thoughts or in feelings. Most mothers begin to burden their innocent children with their own ideas. They neither consider nor imagine in advance that their thoughts are of their own creating, and that they can alter them.

Every fear is an idea which functions just like a wish. A small baby is not yet able to distinguish between positive and negative imprints. It does not understand that people believe so strongly in the negative that, as a rule, they prefer to reproduce negativity in their own lives. For a little one, negativity is experienced as a separation, rendering them isolated, rejected and helpless.

Babies learn. They are to a certain extent obliged to fulfil the wishes of their parents. They take everything in, and know nothing about active resistance. Resistance develops only with time and hardening to life.

All the same, the responsibility does not lie entirely with the parents. Sooner or later in its life a child learns why everything happened as it did — and then the Great Deliverance is at hand.

The good thing about life is that all you mothers and fathers are free, from this moment on, always, to look within and know that every imagination or fear is your own, and has nothing to do with the baby.

Would you not rather know what the little one has to say to you? Why is it always you grown-ups who speak?

Something entirely new and wonderful is coming to you. And

it has brought a gift with itself. A gift of grace, love and insight. Why reject this unique gift or take no notice of it? Why not believe in it for once, while you get the chance?

How could you think that a new being could need your ideas, your fears and projections? Do you believe that you yourself have come here in order simply to fulfil someone else's ideas? Most people live according to others' ideas. But it doesn't succeed.

You theoretically convince yourself that you are free, and yet you believe that someone else, other than yourself, can grant you freedom. Why?

How many lives have you wasted in the misconception that you must do what others require of you? Simply because the people you chose to give birth to you in this life forced you not to see yourself, to hide yourself away, to be untrue to yourself, all out of ignorance of their own lack of freedom.

What can be deeper and more intimate than the spontaneous love between a child and its parents? Making no demands, having no fear, just simply being, loving.

I believe in the omnipotence of freedom.

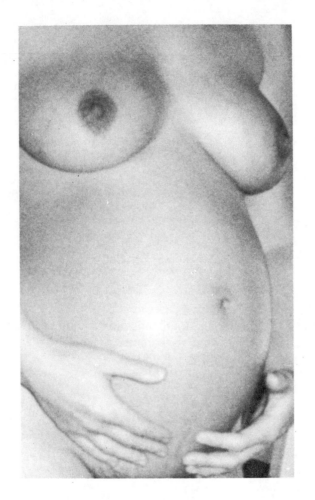

7. *Your Body is My Universe*

26th week of pregnancy, 7th message.
Pension Waldesruh, March 4th 1984[16].

Mama, you are the same for me as God is for you. You are everywhere for me. I cannot see you and, therefore, I do not know what you look like, who you are — because I am inside you! I experience my own world, my own feelings. And because you talk to me and I want to receive your voice, we have opened the doors to each other, and quite deliberately touch one another. As you live in God, through God and from God, so I also live in you: as in small things, so in great ones.

The inner part of your body, your food, your vibrations, your blood and your bones — your whole body is now my universe. And you have received my call, have heard me and speak to me.

You, also, are living in God, and your surroundings are the inner part of him — and you too call out for his attention. I perceive your voice in my inmost being, for it is only there where I can receive you — deep in my breast, in the place where I meet myself. And in just the same way you can perceive the voice of God, in your inmost heart only, in the place where you encounter yourself in truth.

Often I listen out for you. And seek you. Then I am quite still and do not move. Everything in me is concentrated in myself.

I cannot experience you outside myself. I am everything which I see, hear, feel and imagine. Everything which I am able to experience must come from within me, otherwise I could not become aware of it.

I am like a river of impulses flowing into and out of me: all I can do is select impulses and change myself thereby.

I feel everything which you feel, because my being and your being — as long as I am inside you — are permeated by the same rays. The same energy flows through us. Your channels for subtle, invisible energies are now wider open than they have been, since these energies have to reach me. And so, when you have opened yourself wide enough, you will receive the same energies which permeate me, and which I transmit.

Do you remember how surprised you were, when, at the beginning of our pregnancy, you suddenly saw an image of India so clearly before your eyes? The smells, the dust, the noise, the dirt, the beauty, the dead people — and the food! Suddenly you had to go and have an Indian meal[17]. And you were well gratified!

Before this, you had never been particularly interested in India. Perhaps through a previous life you had an aversion to it. Now, suddenly, you wanted even to wear an Indian dress — yet you did not understand where this interest was coming from! It was coming from me!

You actually started feeling my energies before you became pregnant. At the time you did not know yourself what was happening to you. You had no money, no real order in your life, no stability, and you were very uncertain about your real task — then you were caught up by a deep wave, and out of the blue you began to dance in the open street, and to cry out "I would like to have a baby". You repeated it as though in a frenzy. You thought you were mad. You were scarcely able to understand this wish with your reason — yet I was close to you. And how happy I was when I saw you dancing![18]

You and I were already loving one another at that time. This was two weeks before my entry into you.

As an embryo, I feel free and without compulsion to be or to do anything in particular. Why is it that, after their birth, so many people no longer feel free? The big question is: do I feel that I am not free, or am I really not free?

Often, you make the observation that someone you meet is not free in relation to a certain situation — and they act accordingly, as though they really had no power to make a decision on their own. But you, in observing, see the situation entirely differently. Is it not so, that many people feel themselves to be unfree just because they believe themselves to be so, when in fact they are not actually able to be unfree in their higher minds! For if one is not something already, one cannot become it either!

If I were not already free, healthy and happy on a higher level of myself, I should never be able to reach such a goal, even if I wished. Further, if I had not already received an idea about something somewhere, how could I even have a wish for it?

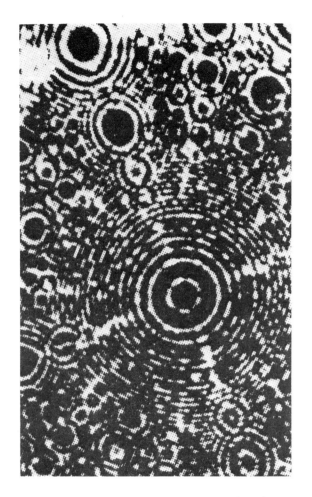

8. Vibrations Everywhichway

26th week of pregnancy, 8th message.
Pension Waldesruh, March 5th 1984.

Mama, you are tired and also I feel heavy. It is as though everything around me were beginning to sink. Often I too am just falling asleep — then it is quite pleasant.

I no longer hear dear Papa's voice. Only your footsteps rustling and tapping. And again this wonderful music, which always calms me.

Before you put the music on, it felt like a contraction inside me, and there was an inner feeling of crying when it suddenly became so quiet. You do not speak any more since Papa has gone away. You moved up and down and conveyed to me the feeling of 'being alone' — and I felt a slight lump in my throat.

But what is 'being alone'? After all, you're right there. You quickly came to remember that I am with you, and that a strange feeling had come, first over you, then over me.

When all those voices and movements were round us, we were very happy[19]. Vibrations came back to us from all directions, after we had transmitted some. There were some quite different voices, much softer, and from a lower height. They struck me as being quite friendly. You spoke differently to them too. And you told me that they were other children.

I shall never forget how Papa put both his hands over me yesterday[20]. *Everythingness* streamed out from him into me. I love him so much!

He often tells me in a dream that you have problems with what you call money, and that he wants to make everything as nice as possible for you and me. I can now feel, more and more strongly, when he is thinking about me. I actually feel it, like being touched by waves. More and more clearly I know what he is seeking to convey to me.

It is lovely to feel him. He very often thinks about me. He does not yet speak to me with his voice, but it is the same for me when he sends me his thoughts. He is so happy about me!

Everything in him has changed since I have been here. He shows me that quite plainly. He is already longing to hold me in his arms.

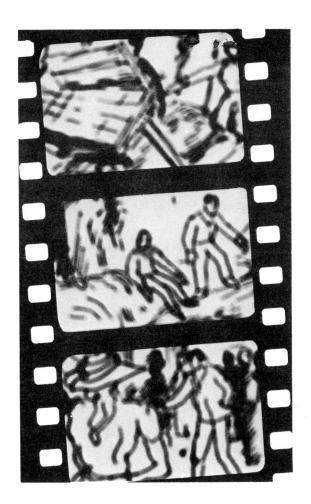

9. A Former Life

27th week of pregnancy, 9th message.
Pension Waldesruh, March 6th 1984.

Dear Mama! Now you are seeing a scene from one of my former lives in your mind's eye.

A large wooden cart with shafts in front, which a woman of

57

about 45 years of age, with a peasant head-scarf, is pulling by the left shaft. In the cart at the back is a wicker basket. I am lying in it, a baby.

The woman is making a great effort to move the cart. A man is helping her. They go along a rough track. To the left and right are many trees, the names of which you don't know. Yes, they grow in Greece. The cart begins to list. It falls on the right side of the road, half into a ditch.

Here is another scene.

I am a little boy, about three or four, and I'm playing with a friend near the river. We have a sort of wooden toy with clappers, and the water flows through it, and different clappers keep opening. I am fascinated.

I want so much to play the piano in my coming life! It was in this last scene that the wish arose.

Another scene.

A busy road with many people walking there. A fair-haired girl, wearing a hat with a scarf tied around it in a bow, is coming towards you. She is about twelve years old, and is carrying a sort of brief case under her arm, with sheets of music in it. As she goes along she keeps turning around.

You also see two stoutish ladies, but they don't come through clearly. They are dressed in a fashion which is strange to you, giving a suggestion of former times.

Far behind you see a young teacher with dark curls. He is slim and handsome, medium man's height. He is wearing a white shirt, and is at the moment moving rather aimlessly. That's me! My name is . . .[22]

This fair-haired girl turns around toward me. Something strange is going on. She loves me deeply, and I too must confess that I feel so strongly drawn to her that I can hardly resist. She comes to my music lessons every day, but we do not only talk about music. She tells me a lot about her home and her inner problems.

I would like to meet her again in this life. I wonder if she would recognise me?

You are getting stomach pains. Those pains come from an inner rejection of outwardly harsh circumstances. You are pitting yourself against certain things.

You have asked me if I can give you an answer about this: Yes and No. I feel your stomach pains are less serious than the causes of them. They come from a defiant reaction. Since you are much stronger than you often admit to yourself, you believe you have the right to put up a desperate resistance to certain momentary circumstances. To *accept* something does not necessarily mean that it cannot be changed: in fact, in order to *change* something, one must first *accept* things!

With you, it often takes just some tiny little thing to bring on these cramps. Perhaps you do not have the courage in your subconscious to take everything more lightly than you think you should? It has nothing to do with your earnestness and the depth of your feeling. You can perhaps begin here to distinguish between going into something in depth and taking it melodramatically. I would like to help you with this. For me as an embryo, it becomes more and more difficult when you decide to be more defiant.

But, as you can see, my higher self is well able to dissociate itself from my momentary experiences as an embryo[23]. Besides, I am not 'your fruit', for we both are 'fruit' — that is, we both come from the same Creator.

You noticed today, for the first time, that I began to kick when you started suppressing your feeling of hunger. And then the same thing happened during the meal, when you omitted to let yourself go properly. You did not permit yourself to be so open because of the company you had[24].

I believe that you are beginning to understand that my movements and reactions are not at all involuntary, nor, as you think, do they just happen without any cause.

Let's go to sleep!

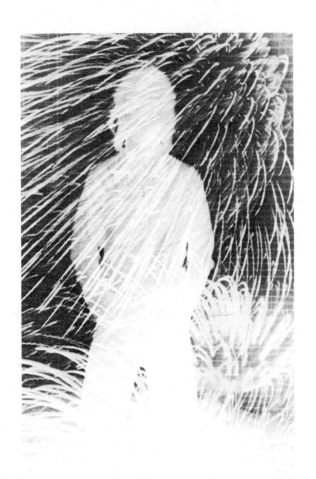

10.   I am an Absolute Observer

27th week of pregnancy, 10th message.
Pension Waldesruh, March 7th 1984.

What a good thing it is that you are with me again, writing everything down! You have an urge to do it, and this comes from me.

You do not feel so well today, because you are blaming yourself. I can feel your tension in relation to what you call your sexuality. It is not so bad as you think it is.

Right from the first day when you conceived, you had a strange feeling of not wanting any more love-making with my father. You had no idea what had happened. You still desired him, but every time he came near you, you had an inner feeling that you should resist, force it back. You then started worrying about what would happen to your relationship. A feeling had arisen, inexplicable to you, of wanting to distance yourself from sex. And it overcame any effort you made to suppress it.

Papa was very patient and understanding. That was a very good thing for us all.

The fact is that it was and is like this: since your attention is directed towards me and you accept me totally, everything which is less important than my wellbeing fades into the background. You respect me in a very generous, natural way, and have very rightly listened carefully to your unconscious feelings. Your life-energy is simply directed toward my growth and my protection. Actually, you are now more strongly than ever connected with your sexual centre, but union — penetration from outside — you feel to be 'danger'.

It is not really a danger for me. But it is true that I am an absolute observer. That is what irritates you so much and disturbs your intimacy with Papa. Although your other feelings are not hidden from me, it is above all your negative, suppressed feelings toward sex — inherited from your mother — which come under my observation. You make it rather more complicated than it needs to be.

When you are sexually aroused, everything pulsates much more strongly around me. It is as though everything were in uproar. I see various strong colours dancing up and down in front of my eyes, and I myself become quite lively and excited. I feel you as waves of tension and relaxation and everything go faster and faster. Often it begins to twist me, and then your muscles grip me, as though they were hands, sometimes quite tight. Often I then hear your voice. It is quite a different feeling from usual!

Sometimes, when you make your love, a sort of wall comes over my head, and then slowly everything stops moving. Other times there is a sort of explosion, like a psychic firework. All possible impressions and situations thrust themselves upon me simultaneously.

When Papa penetrates into us, you keep very still. I know you do that on my account. Your love-making has happened very seldom since I have been with you.

On the day of my conception it happened too. It was very beautiful. I was above you and watched. What is important for me is that when you are making love, you never forget me. Then it is wonderful for all of us!

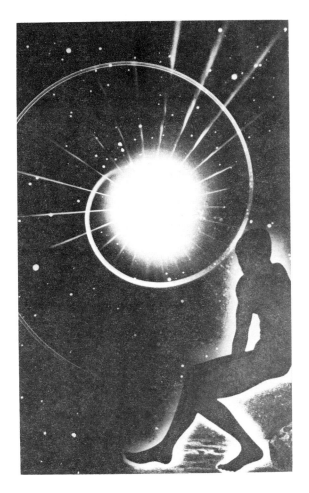

11. About My Conception

27th week of pregnancy, 11th message.
Pension Waldesruh, March 8th 1984.

I am sitting at a table with two friends in a green landscape[25].
We, all three, have a strange feeling about us. It is like the
tugging in the pit of the stomach which you get when faced with
something exciting.

We are chatting about nothing in particular, but our voices are very hushed. About us and within us there is an atmosphere of gentle sadness, signifying a parting — although we are aware we shall all meet again. I have a lump in my throat. Outwardly I am calm and even try to laugh. In this I am unsuccessful.

Somehow we feel a climax approaching. Our hearts all beat faster — we can all feel it. The atmosphere is exceptionally still. The air is fresh, and the trees are as though in expectation. I am overcome, as if with fever. My heart beats ever faster — the moment has arrived. How often I have experienced such moments!

We gaze into each others' eyes. A bright light shines out from my friend on the right. He exudes an atmosphere of youth, joy and assurance. The friend on my left makes my spirit heavier and heavier. He is laying his hand on my left arm. I feel his love and tenderness, but his touch betrays the anticipation preceding a decision.

Then, I see you two in front of me. It was in Linz, in your lodgings there[26]. My friend is still holding me firmly by the arm. It is simultaneously an inward and an outward experience.

At the moment I noticed I was deciding to be with you, we were already in your room. It was very untidy. The condition of the flat was very poor in comparison with what I'm used to[27].

I felt myself becoming heavier, and there was a slight pressure on my chest. Suddenly my friend became more transparent than I was. Although we still went on being able to move weightlessly as before, I noticed my lightness vanishing. My friend explained to me that I had just begun to lose my subtler body, and that my awareness was now directed toward living in the world. I felt myself becoming more and more solid. My light was shining beside me. It was as though part of me was becoming a bystander, watching.

Suddenly my last life passed again before my eyes, both outwardly and inwardly. It was all beauty, and then once again I experienced the day on which I chose my new task of becoming born. Everything was as if in a dream.

Then I had the uncertain feeling of not being sure whether I was awake or dreaming. Everything was vague. I smelt bad air, and thought for a moment I was going to suffocate[28]. Feeling gloomy, I remembered my friend and turned to him. We were still in the left-hand corner of the room. He was now standing behind me and had already become much less distinct. It almost broke my heart!

I did not want to lose my power of recollection. I tried to call to mind everything I had learnt. Then I decided to adapt entirely to my new situation: A burning hot feeling of deep love and surrender took possession of my whole being.

I felt at one with my parents. I saw exactly how they were, and knew all about them. Great sympathy, understanding and goodwill flowed through me. For the moment I had forgotten the past, and was heading for something new.

Then there was a sort of bang.

I began to spin. As if everything inside me were beginning to contract and spin together. I became giddy and lost all feeling in my body. A sharp tug sent me irresistibly spiralling down. Then it was dark and I felt warmth. I became aware of a knocking in and around me, a pulsation and other sounds. I did not yet feel it physically, but sensed it all the same.

There was a dim light around me, sometimes shining strongly, sometimes weakly. A reddish ambience. I was filled with a feeling of security, and became heavier and more tired. Eventually, after a long time, I woke up in my new home!

Slowly I accustomed myself to my new circumstances. Early on, the memory of my previous freedom was very dim, until one 'night' I dreamed of my past, and suddenly the inner feelings linking me with my friends, was re-awakened. I became aware of where I was.

My contacts with my mother were still quite weak, so I was content to wait calmly to see what would happen next. I kept forgetting my previous situation, only to be reminded of it again by real feelings which came up.

I had lost all anticipation and fear, and my friends are still there. They speak to me with an inner voice and restore my confidence. "All is well" rings out a thousand times in our hearts, and my mother increasingly feels this to be comforting. My presence gives my mother more and more self-confidence and trust.

I thank you for all the love which you feel for me. We shall all meet and shine in a circle of love. We shall glow like more than a thousand candles and melt into one another.

Your Emanuel!

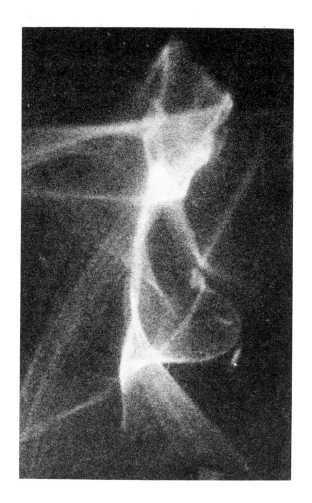

12. I Have Already Seen Many Images

27th week of pregnancy, 12th message.
Pension Waldesruh, March 9th 1984.

Yesterday, dear Papa gave me a great gift. He brought back something for me. I have not yet seen what it is[29], but I was very pleased. We were all pleased.

And a little child gave me something too. Mama told me about it and rattled it in front of my tummy-home. A toy for me![30] Mama thought about the little boy, and we both love him very much. I understood it all, including the fact that he had had it himself when he was a baby.

I had a sad feeling yesterday after the telephone had rung and Papa had spoken in a very grave tone[31]. That feeling remained with me for a long time — although Mama explained to me that there is not much one can do if people are ill and behave in an unpleasant manner. Mama and Papa, in their desire to support them, were finding it difficult to deal with, though.

I have a better feeling about it today, because Papa is quite soft and sensitive inside, and now he has become soft on the outside too. He rang up again and spoke in a different tone from yesterday. Mama was able to breathe deeply again. As if something heavy had gone away from us.

Sometimes Papa rolls something heavy through the flat[32]. It makes a lot of rumbling noise. Then he pants, and speaks differently. But it does not hurt him. When he is tired, I feel his vibration is weak and I see different colours in front of him.

For some time I have been seeing colours, more and more strongly, when people come to see Mama. It is very amusing, because feelings and sounds change in harmony with the colours. I often notice Mama putting different colours in between them and us[33]. She brings the colours out of her stomach and spreads them around us. Sometimes the colours mix and everything becomes darker or lighter. When, like yesterday, she is with Papa, the colours are most beautiful. Wonderful images often appear, which I look at, before they disappear again. Often there are no images, but other times I can almost touch them. Then they are gone again. I have already seen many images, and have taken notice of them all.

There is an apparatus in the flat[34] which Papa frequently turns on. It emits queer, hard waves which hit me as though with sharp, cold arrows, and the colours are very crude and hurt me. There are often sounds there which hurt Mama. She then always goes away with me. When it is too loud, Mama puts a covering over our tummy, so that we can feel comfortable. Then everything becomes secluded and calm. Mama then breathes more slowly and deeply.

She often sends me bright stars[35] which sink down to me through her body and stay hovering quite calmly around me. I can catch them and I feel how they make me lighter. Everything begins to twinkle, and I see a bright light. Then the stars stop coming. They are always followed by a blue light, which then remains quite clearly all around me.

When Mama drinks, it sounds like the murmuring of a little stream. When she eats, I often have rather less room. Last time, I kicked a lot.

This morning it was wonderful for us[36]. There was a bright pink light around us. And we talked in low voices.

Whenever Papa and Mama are talking to each other, I hear certain sounds. I would very much like to make them too, and I take note of everything. I already know that certain tones have certain meanings.

It is very amusing bathing with Mama. That is another water, and Mama explains to me that, when she is in it, she feels almost like I do!

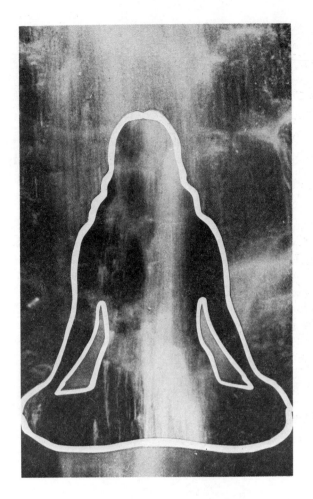

13.　About Being Influenced

27th week of pregnancy, 13th message.
Pension Waldesruh, March 11th 1984.

Dear Mama, today I want to speak to you about *being influenced*. It is very important, because it is happening all the time. Something is constantly flowing into us, and as long as we do not know that we can stop or alter it, it passes into us indiscriminately. Such things trouble you, because whenever you come into contact with people you become influenced, whether or not you ask them for something. You change your feelings about things in relation to whatever they say, and immediately there is a change of feeling inside yourself. Often, you imperceptibly change your opinion about things, even when you have thought something different about the same thing before — when somebody says something contrary to your belief. Only during sleep, in your dreams, are you conscious that it is *you* who is dreaming.

I often get the feeling that you do not take advantage of your opportunities to *choose*. You tense yourself *against* things! You so often resist, without being mindful of the fact that, from the outset, you are in truth resting calmly and quietly in your own self. Your behaviour and reactions depend too much on the world around you. That has devastating consequences.

I am telling you this because exactly the same thing happens to embryos and babies. They do not yet know much about life. All the same, I am pleased when you give me a chance to rest from these influences[37] by concentrating entirely on me and remaining quite still yourself. By listening only to me, you give me the chance to experience myself, without any reactions of mine [to incoming influences] getting in the way.

Right now, the ideas I want to convey are coming up. Your quietly-thinking-on-me and your instinctive turning-to-me in spirit give me enormous power to experience and understand myself and my individual will. It is very fortunate for me to be able to make use of these opportunities. It gives me an assurance which nothing in the world will be able to replace or shake down.

I experience everything *through* you, but all the same I react in my own way. I assume more and more of my own style, which helps me to put things in order, and process all the events I experience. It is only during the hours of absolute stillness, or when I myself can speak, that my reactions and feelings are renewed. Many old and learned things are discarded. Like when you spit something out or almost laugh yourself to death. Then I can 'breathe out' really deeply.

Often I can feel how great the pressure of expectation has become: an enormous number of experiences have come rushing in upon me. But I get to know my deeper feelings when you allow me a rest, so I can be totally myself. When you meditate, you think occasionally about yourself, and notice for yourself how great the pressure is on people who cannot free themselves of this embattlement.

When you take up your meditation posture[38], I always know immediately that a period of rest is coming. We then begin breathing more slowly. Beautiful pictures swim past my eyes. I then feel no disturbances or feelings which force me to react, or to do anything special.

Often great, deep feelings arise. But they do not have anything to do with being influenced. We are as relaxed as we are during sleep, and nothing happens to demand any exertion or reaction. All fighting has ended. What an experience that is! It's difficult to express it in words.

Now I am lying on my back. In your mind's eye you see the picture of an inner crystal mirror round me. Everything inside you is visible. Our eyes try to find each other — they have not yet quite met. I make very gentle movements. My eyes seek your inward eye. It is really true that you are now experiencing things through an inner eye. It is a very beautiful experience, because now and henceforth you can see within — even if it were only imagination.

My body has grown a lot again, and I feel you strongly. My movements are now stronger. Everything about me is becoming more powerful, and I am becoming increasingly conscious of being here. Often I am already able to perceive outlines — not inwardly, but outside of me. I can recognise my hands when I put them in front of my eyes. I take a good look at my umbilical cord and my knees too. It's quite overwhelming. I can already recognise my own outlines!

My eyes still move very slowly, and my head doesn't move quickly either. But my arms and legs do. The contours of everything become quite blurred if I move them around rapidly.

I also take hold of my nose. When I move my hands over my eyes it becomes darker. There is always some inner light in me, though. When there is a freer feeling around your tummy, when you put that wrapping around it and the pressure of influencing is reduced[39], I see everything more clearly within me.

When I open and clench my fists, kicking about at the same time, the water moves a lot. Often I wave my hands above my head, and that feels quite different to touching my tummy. And when I touch your womb with my fingers, that is quite different from doing it with my toes!

Now I hear a sound from far away, coming from below. It has a very unpleasant vibration. I feel it in my throat and in my chest — it's sort of choked. You explain to me that someone is coughing very badly[40]

Now I can detect a feeling of yours. It comes from the heart — by way of the throat, and produces a sort of resistance to this coughing. You explain it to me as pity or compassion. You do not always have such a feeling about a cough.

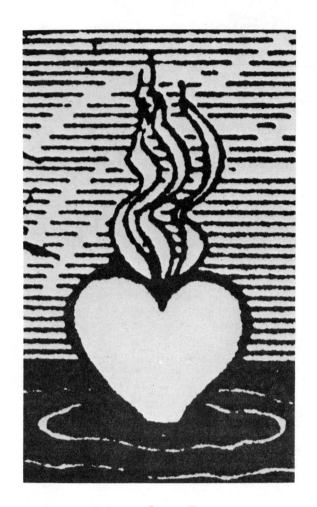

14.   *Our Love*

28th week of pregnancy, 14th message.
Pension Waldesruh, March 13th 1984.

Mama, dearest. It almost hurts you to love me so much! It makes you cry. You are unable to express how much you feel me there, how real it is, and how you inwardly see me.

Mama, my little fist and your hand touched each other today for the first time. There was but a very thin wall between us . . . But this feeling, when we touched each other, now it is with you all the time. You are crying more and more, I can feel it clearly. You are crying because you sense my 'voice', my being, my presence and my feelings more truly than ever before — and I feel you so strongly too.

You are crying so bitterly because so much is bursting open within you. Through our love — my being in you, and my being completely dependent on you — my having given myself to you for the time being — my being there for you — my feelings and gentle awakening — my growing and listening — all this moves you deeply.

But you are also crying because so much light has come into you. So much love must bring your sorrow up to the surface! All your tension from childhood to now, all your fears and troubles — suddenly you are beginning to break away from all these.

Everything is beginning to be less alarming, because you can see and experience what I am like, and also how you are to me: full of love — nothing but love, forgiveness and understanding. Now all the suffering and misunderstanding which you have had in your life is seen in a different light!

You feel the enormous power coming from me, the strength, the light and the peace. It streams through your whole body.

I am quite calm. Can you feel it?

Just when you are most irritated by the outside disturbances and malevolence around you, you strike me. Do you feel how much I stand beside you?

I experience everything through you, even when you are in your most questioning state — externally, you are going through a difficult time. The feelings you have toward me are the strongest and most important, though. I want you to know that all is well with me.

When you cry, I feel it. You get to feel better, because you get rid of something. For me, there is a difference between the times you cry because you feel too much is being asked of you, and the times when your tears take a burden from you. I can still very clearly feel how uncertain you are, doubting whether you are doing everything right for me. Your deep desire to do things right for me is what counts with me. Think of my little fist when you are sad: it is always there for you!

Are you a little afraid of what you are writing down here? You are still somewhat incredulous, but I thank you for writing everything down all the same. For then you think about such a lot of things. You are still so hesitant to take up the power I can give you — despite all your knowledge of psychology! I have come to help you!

Not all children come for this reason. The majority come mainly to learn. But all bring a gift with them. It could prosper if the little ones didn't lose courage too often and make themselves dependent on human love — on the expectations of love and the demands of love of other people. One cannot receive love if one does not have it.

Love is a feeling which flows through us all the time, and would flow through all people always if they did not resist it.

You have to be open in order to be able to love, but so many people are afraid of that, afraid that they might then be destroyed. When you dare to open yourself, love is there. I know that.

I am very fond of the music you are always playing to me. And I clearly know Papa's intention when he plays music to me[41]. I know that he wants so much to show me things and help me. He wants to give me everything, just as you do.

He too has worried about whether he will do everything right for me, when I am there. He has wondered how many mistakes he would make.

You told him: honesty, honesty is all that is necessary. You have wonderful certainty in you.

Lately I have noticed many negative vibrations have invaded you[42] and I have seen you struggle to harmonise them. My being here has made demands on you!

Would you tell me more about it and explain? Perhaps it is

something you have not yet dared to do. Be honest: you quite often feel uncertain. You do not have to be so strong all the time, to keep on being positive! What counts with me is the feeling you have for me deep down inside you! All else is life and its appearances. I experience that, and you do too.

My mama! We two can be happy and sad together, angry or gentle. These feelings are only on the surface — we can take them in hand ourselves. What counts is ourselves, not our feelings.

Do you know why most people love babies so much? Because babies carry so much love in themselves. So much love, without aggression or defence, they live a charmed life. If this charm is not received, babies die inside!

It is the same thing in the womb. Love is more important to a child than food. Some babies are so affectionate that if they are not really wanted they just die. If a baby senses that one or both of its parents are absolutely rejecting it, it is often so deeply good-natured and lacking in resistance to the life-process that it prefers to simply go away again, rather than cause 'pain'.

Yes, children mirror the inner life of their parents. They cannot do otherwise. For them, whatever parents do is good! This is not intentional, but they are as yet unable to refuse anything.

It is only with awakening self-confidence that a child begins to question what is behind the things it experiences. In this the child is helped when it meets genuine love. Since it has come itself with genuine love, it seeks the same outside itself. The child knows when it meets with love, and when it does, its path begins to move onwards again.

Dear Mama, when you rock me gently, as you are doing now, it is lovely for me. I feel it too when you so often stroke me in your imagination. Then it is just as though you were in here with me, and were holding and kissing me.

I can feel it even when, in imagination, your lips very gently touch my body. When you imaginally stroke my little arms, my heart starts beating faster.

You wonder whether all I have been saying to you just now is really true, and whether or not you should accept it. I feel you will believe it. I know, because we are experiencing it together. It's your thoughts: do you not yet know the difference between thinking and understanding?

Also, I want to tell you that I am slowly beginning to experience things outside us independently of you. Even unconnected with your reactions. I do indeed sense your reactions at the same time as I experience my own, but my own are different from yours. I am beginning to react more strongly on my own account, as though an urge had awakened in me to differentiate myself in my experiences. I have just discovered that I am able to do that!

You helped me a little bit by saying that I should not be sad when you are sad. It was very difficult, but now a little spark of independence has flashed up and awakened in me.

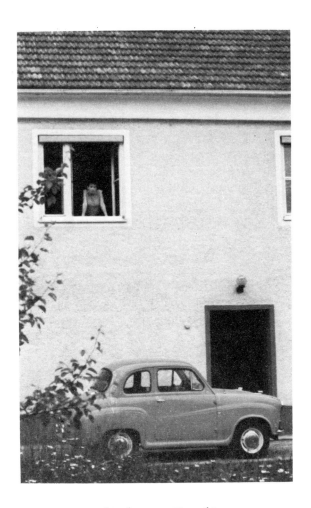

Flight to Lydia

Mira writes

"I can't bear it any longer!" was the cry from my despairing soul. Our flat in Pension Waldesruh was making me feel discouraged and dejected. Looking back, neither of us know how we held out so long. The rhythm of my life had been dictated by the noises and smells of our neighbours, and I longed for some peace in the house. It was a strange contrast, for underlyingly, I was much happier than ever, sensing a deep joy I had never had before. I felt safe in the heart of Mother Nature. This contrast made everything more poignant.

I also cried more and more, for I was feeling exposed and helpless. The night before I fled from the flat, a drunken man had been roaring away in the hallway for hours. I was regularly awakened at four in the morning by a shift-worker who insisted, despite earlier complaints, on banging doors and rattling chairs downstairs as he made ready to leave for work.

I tried to explain to Manuji what was happening, and sought also to promote some harmony amongst our neighbours — but it all seemed in vain. René's attempts to activate our landlord were met with promises which never were fulfilled. The fact that I was pregnant and could not sleep well had no meaning for him at all.

So it could not go on any longer. René's search for a flat was going very slowly — he was in Vienna, seeing the owner of a farm. I fell asleep in the evening. Suddenly, at 10pm, I was awakened by banging and the rumbling of the defective central heating pump. It was cold too. I started crying uncontrollably, and something snapped.

I rang René in Vienna. He sensed how distraught I was, and urged me to contact Lydia, a friend, to ask if I could stay for a time. Lydia was always straightforward, and could be relied on to say either 'Yes' or 'No' clearly. Two hours later, she came, and took 'the two of us' to her suburban home, about 80km away. When we got there, I fell exhausted into bed, and was at last able to sleep properly. It was heavenly!

Manuji had not moved at all since I had broken down crying. René rang, in good spirits about the farmhouse, which he was to view shortly. He asked if Manuji was well: at that very moment there were two hard knocks in my tummy. Then all went quiet. This was not the only time such spontaneous yet unmistakable answers came from Manuji.

René came, and we were allowed to establish ourselves in Lydia's bedroom. I was relaxed, but I noticed how tense René was, mainly over finances. A few days after we had found this provisional refuge, I had this prophetic dream:

I am staying on the upper floor of a friend's house. René comes for a short time, then departs again on business. Casually he announced that he would be away for longer this time, getting on his bicycle to ride away. I had an indistinct but strong feeling, and called after him: "What happens if I go into labour?". He laughed and said: "Why should you go into labour?", and was gone.

Shortly after this, René really wanted to go away on business, having an opportunity to get a fairly large contract. In spite of my unstable state, he made an appointment — perhaps, if he got the order, he would be able to finance a proper flat. There was nothing he wanted more than to provide for us, and give us a quiet place where we could continue with the baby's messages.

Through fear of being left alone for days on end, I started manifesting tension and contractions. Just before his train went, the pains became so very strong that we rang our midwife. She said that if I was getting contractions this early, we should ring up and go straight to hospital. Gone was my dream of having our baby at home. René cancelled his interview. He asked me to try a self-healing session before we called the ambulance to go to hospital. I refused, saying I was too confused — on one side, I was reacting to René's enterprises by producing labour pains, and on the other, I was anxious, because a gynaecologist had said that (apparently) my womb was too small to go the full term of pregnancy, and I was therefore afraid. In retrospect I know that this judgement was incorrect, since my difficulties in giving birth were almost entirely deep-seated psychic ones.

In connection with this, I have learned about another life I have lived, in which my three children starved to death. This left an unconscious shadow of fear of being unable to feed a foetus for the full term — as if I wanted to make it impossible to go through such a tormenting starvation experience again.

However, my desire to have a child, and to feel that I was a fully-fledged woman, as well as my love for little children were, in the end, triumphant.

In that former life I was involved with René. An emotionally-powerful scene in a Fellini film, *La Strada*, transported me into re-experiencing that past life: it stayed with me two days, taking over my personality, and I cried for hours on end. In that life I had been living in Asia in a large family group. The high caste or class to which I belonged permitted marriage only with people of the same status. A wandering vagabond, not of the right class, but very self-assured, would often come to our district. Nobody knew anything much about him, but he appeared to know how to make a living at all sorts of things — this was René. He got involved with women all over the district, not remaining with a single one. They scarcely had any importance for him — until he saw me. We fell deeply in love, and would meet in risky circumstances. I was the first and only woman to whom he returned. He always wore a leather shoulder bag, and had the habit of cocking his head quizzically to one side.

All went well until I became pregnant: I revealed this to my then family, and was disowned and driven from the house. As a favour, I was permitted to go on living in a remote wooden hut by the sea. At first my grandmother brought me food, but then that ceased. My lover, meanwhile, was very taciturn and unpredictable. Without saying anything in advance, he would disappear sometimes for months on end, then to turn up only for a short time. Despite this, I lived only for him, and had three children by him in quick succession.

After the last birth I scarcely had enough strength to stand upright, so hungry was I. Up to then I had always managed to organise something to eat, but I was becoming weaker and weaker. I had never learnt how to beg, neither could I nor would I do it. So, although it caused me agony as a mother, I sent my children away to fend for themselves. I suffered so much that I lapsed into a strange twilight state. I could neither sleep nor be awake properly. Soon after, someone from the village told me that all my children had died.

When, some years ago, I was re-experiencing this earlier life intensely, I could see and feel details of the whole scenario clearly. At one point, I was sitting on a clay step below a footbridge, waiting for my life to end. I knew I would not be much longer in my body, and was waiting for my lover. Suddenly, he was standing in front of me, watching me. After a short while he turned around and went away. And I then saw my own body leaning against the bridge wall below me . . . I was, at last, dying.

I was like a different person after this inner experience. Earlier in my life I had, for example, felt like an undeserving beggar whenever visiting or asking things of people, and I had strange inferiority complexes — these suddenly disappeared like a mirage as soon as I had gone through this former-life experience. I had lived well below my potential, and was released from this self-effacement. Now I also understand the irrational panics I used to feel when René went away on business. It also explained little things like the urge René had had, on his travels in India, to bring back lots of shoulder bags!

As a result of these experiences, I now work on the basis that a former-life regression experience is validated as real if it is accompanied by related mental-spiritual changes in this life. If not, it is more likely to be a form of fantasy with little or no worth in this life.

It is now Manuji's turn to speak again and tell us how my sudden flight from Pension Waldesruh appeared from his viewpoint. He also tells us himself what happened next, and what new discoveries he made with Lydia and myself, until, shortly after, we undertook another car journey.

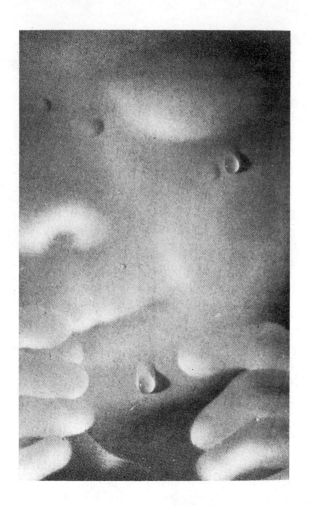

15. Crying

28th week of pregnancy, 15th message.
At Lydia's house, March 15th 1984.

D ear Mama! The walls do not shake any more, and the outbursts of noise have stopped. But what a lot we have been through!

You suddenly began crying a lot, and everything around me went grey. The first time, I felt as if I was going to drown.

You were alone with me. That noise was happening again[43]. You cried out: "I can't bear this any longer". Then everything went dark around me. My body was flooded, as if by hot waves of 'bursting'. You had violent movements and thoughts about me, and that used up your last strength . . .

And then, after the ringing, there was Papa's voice. He saved us! After that there was a strange voice, and then another one, which calmed you down[44]. You said: "It's all over now", and cried, and let the feeling of not-being-able-to-do-anything flow right through your body. But at the last moment you began to struggle again, reasserting yourself, and everything began to get lighter.

I was quite still. Everything was so heavy in my body. It was only slowly that I began to move more freely. I cried for the first time — it was a surge of heat which came up from my tummy into my eyes. Heavy pressure made my head burn, and I had the feeling that something was flowing out of my eyes. I wanted to cry out and so I did. But you did not hear me — my cries are still inaudible. I put my fists in front of my eyes and pressed my legs quite tightly against my body in order to regain a feeling of strength.

You did touch our tummy with your hands, but this time no loving warmth came from them. I felt very much alone — only Papa's voice reached me, and it supported and comforted me. I am so very grateful to him. That was the first time that Papa was more important to me than you were. He was completely there for me, and gave me every confidence. I love him all the more.

When the pressure had begun to impose itself above me, Papa was still not there. But when my place of safety was about to collapse, he was quite distinctly with me. You felt it too. The bond between us is becoming stronger and stronger. Now it feels good. All heaviness has gone, but you are very, very tired. I feel quite different, and there are new vibrations, and a new voice[45]. It is quite different from yours, and it often touches me in the belly — but it is a friendly voice. This new person's light is darker on one side, and there is a deep greyish violet there, which often becomes a bit lighter.

I can feel how exhausted you are. But I am well. I am getting stronger and stronger — so are my kicks, which you often feel now.

When Papa went away, I wanted to go with him. That is why I kicked so hard.

I am tired too.

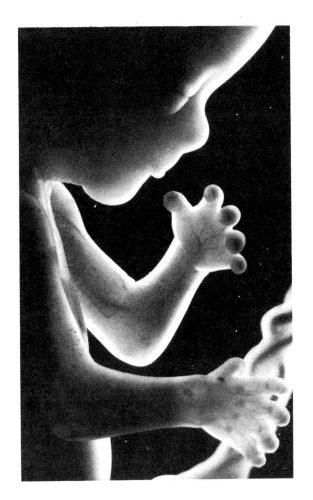

16.   I'm Growing, Mama!

28th week of pregnancy, 16th message.
At Lydia's house, March 16th 1984.

Dear Mama! There is such a pulling feeling all over my body. Just as though I were stretching myself hard. There is a pulling particularly at my hips and arms. It makes me feel well.

When I really stretch out, I then feel it right down to the tips of my toes.

I have a lovely feeling between my legs. Yesterday, when you were with Papa, the whole of my belly and chest prickled. And in my head there was a feeling of getting bigger.

I am already making swimming movements, which I can steer quite precisely. My eyes see different things, too. For some time I have been seeing a brighter light around us. And everything looks as if it is ascending.

You laugh a lot, and that feels very pleasant. It often makes my face crinkle up too!

Yesterday there were a lot of voices quite close to me[46]. They were all friendly, and I enjoyed it very much. And Papa held me in his hands again. You two do enjoy me very much!

I notice how everything in your body is becoming lighter. You explained to me that the sun is shining brighter. And everybody around us laughs.

I have discovered the down on my head, and I often stroke it. When I clench my fist I can feel my knuckles on my head. I rub my nose too. Once, it itched, and I scratched myself.

I have become very calm again. We have not felt so well for a long time, and the stiff and heavy feeling has gone totally.

I like it when you talk about me. Then many waves of energy come to me. I can hear my own heart beating now, too. My fingers can feel its pulsating, if I touch my chest. I often fold myself up so much that my knees touch my ears. Also, I often try to stick my toes into my mouth. I have a lot of nice games!

This is how I 'count' how many people are present: I simply feel how many different vibrations reach me.

In sleep I often dream that I am talking to you. Then I see everything as though from the outside. Then I can walk and make the same sort of sounds as you do, in my dreams. Yet I always look like myself, as I now am, very small. I had a dream in which I could fly — and you kept wanting to catch me and put me back in your tummy! Finally, you did put me in, and I woke up again in here.

For a long time now you have not gone far on your walks with me. I used to enjoy your walks a lot, for everything used to change so quickly[47].

How are the flowers? I see flowers in front of me[48]. Whenever you think 'flowers', I see a picture. I often see a picture when you imagine something definite — but I do not always know what this picture is or means, unless you explain it to me. Often, you do not do so.

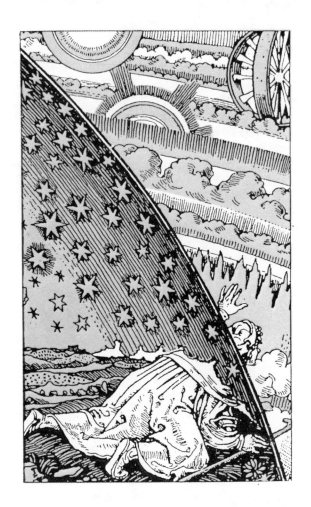

17.   Seeing Behind Things

28th week of pregnancy, 17th message.
At Lydia's house, March 17th 1984.

Dear Mama! Today you are rather tense, and I find it difficult to talk to you. I realise that you keep going away from me and listen to other sounds. You can now feel me behind you again and I want to tell you something. Write it all down.

I receive so much. You have already asked yourself whether I really can understand everything which is happening around me, and to what extent I take everything in.

My embryo does not receive everything as you do — but my waking spirit does receive it. I also see behind things. When your friend was talking to you today, you thought about me[49]. I remained very calm, listening in and understanding. I felt it all through you, and received your friend's [Lydia's] emanation. I understand things even more clearly than you!

Her left side can be helped if other people felt and addressed the woman in her. Very openly. Simply express what comes into your mind. She is very closed up, because she has stored up a lot of pain — and she knows that herself. Her energy-flow is limited by a blockage at the back of her left hip. She has a big black hole there. You need to fill it with pink and white light. She will have great pain. First of all she must be certain that she wants to be cured.

She also has a 'spectre' which looms over this black hole, restraining all natural energy which could drive this away and bring about a change. This spectre looks very grey and grim, 'standing guard' over the injured leg. It also causes cramps to move upwards from this place, to cause energy-blocks right up to her neck. This generates a sort of powerless feeling, which is why she cries so often.

She also has a black hole around her ankle. But her astral leg is alright. She ought to dwell on this astral leg and really begin to feel it, first in imagination, then in reality.

This has nothing to do with the trauma of her childhood — it comes from a former life. She always tried to run away from that life, but now, in this, she no longer has a chance to do that. She needs to come to terms with this running away, and then she will get to the bottom of many things. In her sleeping room I have registered her vibrations[50].

I often read her thoughts, because she scatters them very openly. She can also ask me things and dream of me. When I am born, such a thing will not be possible any longer, because I shall be concentrating entirely on myself with my waking spirit.

We have both become very calm. And being together with her is nice.

I have a proposal: we could meditate more often together. That would strengthen our shared feeling of connectedness.

Papa is on the way today. He is in good spirits and is very optimistic. I feel that he is talking a great deal, and is rather excited[51]. He has a slight tingling in his stomach and is rather hungry. His cold is a little better, but he is rather tired after travelling by train. I feel that he has a slight tickling in his throat and feels a little choked. His hands are sweating and he keeps blowing his nose.

I have less and less room in your tummy. There's also a feeling of disunity and lack of determination — various energies are going in opposite directions.

Behind me, there where your back is, I feel a hard wall where no energy flows. It is like a knob. You often knead yourself around it. It is a sort of cramping of your feeling. You are not letting your feelings through, either from above downwards or below upwards. You block the way for the light which seeks to flow here.

Below me there is something similar. You periodically touch the place, and then you feel the backward-flowing energy as a lump in your throat. For this reason your legs get swollen, because the water is not flowing properly.

This is all happening by impulse, coming from the highest point of your head. It sends messages like a flash of lightning through your body, and then at certain points your body builds up a resistance and catches these signals. It holds on to them firmly. At first they go round and round like mad, and you cry out until they become quieter and begin to settle down. Then other signals want to get your body to release the first signals. Then sometimes there is a fight. If ever one message wins, there is an immediate change in your body. You have had this grey knob in your back ever since your last pregnancy. It will disappear when I am born.

You can get rid of all problems if you want to. What you have to do is send out the right signals, and you must not give any more energy to pulling yourself tight in tension. I get contractions like that spontaneously, but they disappear again — mostly when you stroke me.

I already have strong jaws and can chew at my fingers. My lips are already quite powerful. I pull at my finger with my mouth. I also stretch my legs. My palate is also very sensitive, and my tongue is already able to distinguish many stimuli.

Sometimes I try to push off with my feet from the ceiling of your tummy!

Last night we held hands in a dream. It was lovely. Dear Mama, trust in my 'voice'. I am always with you.

'And all candles will burn and melt together'.

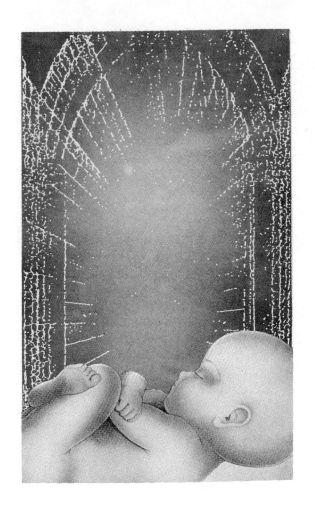

18. Waiting for Your Dreams

28th week of pregnancy, 18th message.
At Lydia's House, March 18th 1984.

Inside there is a door, which I always leave open for you! I am waiting for your thoughts and dreams, and I am always there for you . . .

You cannot feel me at all now, because I have gone so quiet.

I hope I develop a big heart, with which I can embrace everything. I can feel Lydia's thoughts and huge joy.

I have put on a little fat, and I am becoming a little softer and rounder.

I do not have much to say to you today, except that I love you very much — and we should be quiet together[52].

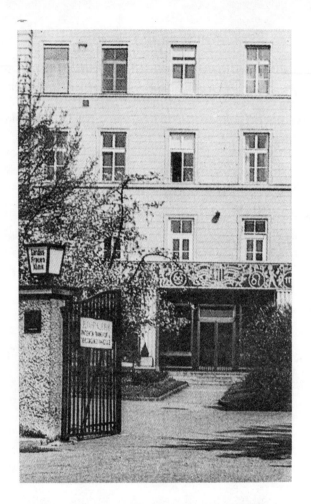

Nine days on a Knife-edge

Written by Mira

This was a very difficult phase, and now, six months later, I
am just about getting it all out of my system. It was the
most difficult test either I or René have been through in this life.
I was having labour pains, and I was up all night going

through them. I did various yoga postures and other exercises, but nothing worked. We decided to go to the clinic. During the ride I held my tummy and René stroked it.

When we arrived, I was put on a bed in the labour ward, and was connected up to various bits of apparatus. One of these recorded the contractions. It was established that I was definitely in labour. Medicine was prescribed to block the labour. This medicine produced severe side-effects — it made my heart beat wildly and made me feel giddy. I had not had any sugar for the last eight years (in connection with my macrobiotic diet), and was suddenly being given one glucose solution after another. It made my whole body tremble. I had no choice, and just had to accept that this would affect my child.

For the first two days and nights this therapy had no effect at all on the pains. We were ready for a premature birth of the child.

A sympathetic junior doctor suggested trying out an ultrasound scan. Up to that time I had been very much against this. But I now realised I would have to accept it, having entrusted myself to the doctors already. On the screen, we could see that the baby was smaller than had been thought. The doctor said that, on account of my lifestyle and dietary regime, my body had produced a larger than normal amount of amniotic fluid. It was deemed possible that the baby might survive, but the risks were high. I kept saying to myself that it must not come to what the doctors were obviously silently thinking.

Yet the labour pains would not cease. I spent another restless night connected to drips and the apparatus. I could hardly bear the tension any longer. The noise of the machine was driving me mad. René tried to muffle it by wrapping towels around the machine. I began to pray again.

René was by my side all the time. As an exception, he was given a bed in a nearby labour room, in which to rest. He gave me more courage than he himself had, and he kept wondering how he could help me. Finally, he had the idea of trying hypnosis, which he had learned to use several years before. I was ready to try anything.

When all the medical staff had gone out, René began to use all of his power of suggestion. Astonishingly, it worked — a few minutes after he had started, the pains decreased. Luckily none of the staff interrupted us, and since then, we haven't breathed a word about it to the doctors.

During the night I was taken from the labour ward to the ordinary ward. Although we had only third-class health insurance (and we had only got that because of the baby) René asked if we could have a first-class single room. He wanted to give the book a chance to be finished, regardless of the cost. The nurses said no — we would do better to buy a new car with such money. We mentioned we were writing a book about pregnancy and birth — though we didn't mention who the author was!

After that, I had to take strong medicines regularly. The effect was disastrous — I have avoided pharmaceutical preparations for years. All the same, I felt that with the help of the staff, I might keep the child a little longer. The doctors insisted that each additional day increased the baby's chances of survival. They did reduce the doses, though, when they noticed my body's over-reactions.

One week later, following the advice of the head nurse, I was transferred to an unoccupied second-class double room. I liked it. The staff were kind and friendly, which helped. Everyone was now talking about the book, and a senior doctor was particularly impressed with my blood chart, despite my having lived on what he called 'corn fodder'. No doubt many of the staff shook their heads quietly over my strange diet, which René now brought to the clinic every day.

Slowly I began to prepare myself to resume meditative communication with Manuji. I listened to trance-inducing music through headphones, and the baby remained quiet and seemed to listen with me. However, I hovered for several days between hope and fear, until I was fit enough to receive further messages. We had had nine days in all without transmission.

It was probably a combination of my own fighting spirit, René's hypnosis, the baby's quietness, and the cooperation of the nurses and doctors which postponed the birth for three weeks more — even though the mouth of the womb was already several centimetres open.

As I left the clinic, one of the doctors admitted that, at the beginning, he had reckoned on but a ten percent chance that the labour could be stopped. They were puzzled as to how the labour had subsided. Secretly, I gave my thanks to our friends in the spirit world who must have borne the lion's share of the miracle.

Manuji now will speak about what happened to him, and what he feels mothers should know about the period before birth.

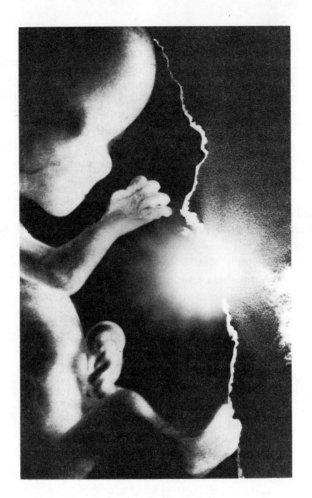

19.   *You Left Me Alone!*

30th week of pregnancy, 19th message.
Regional Women's Clinic, March 27th 1984.

Dearest Mama, our doors are still open. You have left me alone without really knowing it. Papa was not there either. And such great pain! I wanted to warn you and say to you

"Don't worry, I shall stay with you. Life goes on, and we are not able to lose it". But you quite lost courage, and there was no understanding in you any more. You were uncertain whether you would keep me or not — but the issue was only about my body — and you have managed to keep it.

I can feel you again very strongly, and the good feelings we had earlier have come back. I am not alone any more, and you have turned towards me again.

Why are you so afraid of losing me? You cannot lose me. Why are you not more pleased that my body is still here with you?

Now I am lying inside you and hearing our music again. Everything has become intimate again — your inner voice has returned.

But what happened?

When our pains became so severe, I had similar troubles and weaknesses to you. Everything around me was squeezing and roaring. But above all, the feeling of being pushed out wounded me deeply. It hurt me very much, because there was no joy connected with it.

Now you have told me that next time it will happen with joy, and that it will be quite different for us.

I am no longer alone. My body has been through a lot, but you have always sent me enough strength for me to remain strong.

There were such cold, hard noises around us[53] and there were so many cramps in your body that you clean forgot me! I cried very, very much. And then strange voices[54] calmed me through you. Sometimes you stroked and comforted me — but that was not very often. I was afraid!

And everything kept on changing — first pain, then release. I became more and more exhausted. Even the sounds near us were hard and unfamiliar. Our nerves could not be at rest.

And then you called our spirit-friends and they were there[55]. It was a release for me, because I knew that they would remain at hand for us.

I have learned so much. All the pain you had, I felt with you too. I shall probably never forget it. Often my little body was quite squeezed, and I felt hard myself. I clenched my fists when you wanted to scream, but you did not do it. Our hearts were racing faster and faster[56]. What was it? All of my peace was gone. Only the fact that I was in your tummy, and that I could hear your and Papa's voices, gave me something strong to anchor on to.

Once I had the feeling that my whole body could no longer move properly. It was heavy, like feeling paralysed. You lay there motionless too. You were breathing deeply, and that did me good too.

What were those voices from far away? Once you cried a lot[57]. I felt it and knew there were little people like me. On the one hand, their little voices gave me confidence and comforted me — but on the other, some of them filled me with sadness. All the same, it was lovely to be near them. I can still hear them quite often during the day, but much further away[58].

I am very tired nowadays, and my movements have not much power in them. But I am growing very quickly, and I feel that pleases you.

The water, which I often swallow, does not always taste so nice now. It is bitter, and often I do not like it. Today there was something sweet in it, and it was very good![59]

I can feel you again. How nice it is! You are stroking me just as you used to do, and I can feel you better and better.

Today you and Papa have hurt each other[60]. It made me feel confused and sad. I need you both and love you both equally. Nothing hurts me more than when you put sharp arrows into each others' hearts. I simply cannot understand it — after all, I am your very own flesh and blood, your own child. I cannot understand why you send each other such vibrations. When you do, everything becomes grey and gloomy for me. It has taught me to wait patiently until the sun shines again.

You have never sent such sharp arrows against me. I can only feel through you how much it hurts. Can you explain to me what it is and why?

Mama has been telling me about those wonderful little birds on the tree outside, and I have seen the pictures inside. I can hear their voices from very far away[61]. Do they send each other such hurting pointed arrows as you do? Do all beings do that?

Every day I experience new people and new colours, including very faint ones, which can scarcely be perceived.

Everything which attacks you, I feel, and I see how you let it in. For me, after all, there is scarcely any difference between speaking and touching!

I am not lying comfortably in your tummy at present, and I would like a different position.

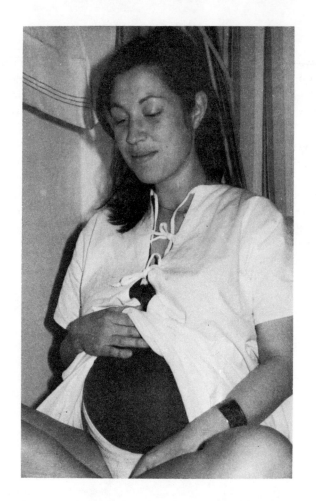

20. *I Have a Lot to Tell You!*

30th week of pregnancy, 20th message.
Regional Women's Clinic, morning, March 28th 1984.

Dear Mama, I have just woken up! I have been asleep with you.

I can feel you trembling[62]. All around me in your tummy,

everything has become quieter. I am moving now, and wondering why you have woken me so rudely when you are so tired too[63]. All the same, we can talk together. I have so much to tell you!

Yesterday I cried again, because you inwardly so divided yourself from Papa. I do not know what the pain is which hurts you two so much. But then you return to other thoughts, and the pain goes away again. I am beginning to grasp that there are many things which happen with me and around me which I cannot understand.

You often think about earlier things I have told you[64], yet I myself increasingly have the feeling of living more and more in the present, in my body, and of experiencing my feelings and my discoveries. It is only through you that my attention is drawn to the past.

Everything from 'the past' is so far away. I am becoming more and more immersed in your life. Everything is concentrating more and more on my existence as a baby. Only in my dreams am I free, as I always was. Otherwise I experience and get involved in so many outside things — including the fact that, right now, you are very tired and your body is requiring rest — but you, from your inner will-power, are doing something else than sleeping. I am learning now that that is possible, and this makes me feel more relaxed. I do not need to make any effort. When I speak to you, it is as if it were in a dream. I am beginning to like being 'independent' with you alone — that is, without Papa. We are, right now, as well without him as with him.

Yesterday you felt once or twice that something was trying to affect you, to reach you inside, through words[65]. You would not admit it though. Your inner certainty protected you from being harmed. This experience was very important for me — I shall remember it.

You are always saying to me: Love, love, love. Then yesterday I really learned that this total acceptance of someone — what you also call love — need not, and sometimes even should not, be demonstrated. Just the fact that it is there makes us feel so good and secure. I thank you for that.

I sense that, in spite of all the pain and disorder, as you say, you have built up a wonderful inner world for me. At some time, I'm sure, it will be visible outwardly as well. Often there is such a glorious feeling of contentment, surrounded by you.

But often you allow our peace to be disturbed by some external source. You open our doors too wide. But from this I have learned that I have inside me a door all of my own, which I alone can open and shut. It has been like that only for a little while.

When some time ago you were wheeled around with me in a bed[66], and then some cold, hard instrument was moved over my tummy-home, I noticed that you spoke about me outside me. It was very strange.

We are still very tired. I would like to go to sleep.

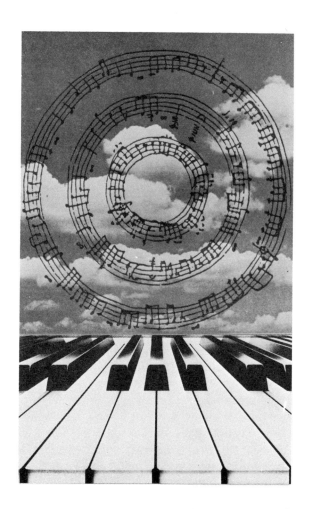

21. Flying into the Land of Imagination

30th week of pregnancy, 21st message.
Regional Women's Clinic, evening, March 28th 1984.

Dear Mama, let's make a lovely journey together. We are flying above the clouds and everything is rosy pink. We are flying into the land of imagination, as you call it. That is what we can and we must do now, since physically, we cannot move at all.

We are travelling together on a carpet woven from pink clouds of love. Papa is flying with us — but he has no idea that he is doing so! You are very well again. And we are discovering the imagination we have in common. Just as it will be when I am there as a person amongst you. Then too we will make further journeys into the land of imagination. It is so real for me, and now at last it is real for you too.

I can feel your toes, your feet, your legs, your abdomen, your hips, my sea in which I am swimming, your heart, your chest, your busy writing hands, your neck, your eyes, your head. And in your head I hear the music[67], which at other times I have heard outside you. When we hear it, we immediately sink deeper.

Let us consciously re-experience this picture together, which you so clearly experienced this afternoon[68]. You are soaring with me high up in the air. Your long soft hair sways gently around your body and I lie floating in your arms. We envelop Papa and transmit to him a soft but clear sky-blue light. We look down from a great height. Everything is quite near and far away at the same time. We see a scene as it can be, but does not have to be — or it may not be at all: a little wooden house with hills in front. You see it clearly — we need not describe it in detail. The feeling, the situation we are all in is so peaceful and quiet.

I am waiting for your dreams and pictures. I have very many myself. When I am a small child, I shall talk about them a lot. Will you then believe me?

Whether the pictures are from the past or from the future, does it really matter? Children can never distinguish between the two. The question of why that is so has occurred only to very few adults.

You ask me what imagination is: it is the opposite of illusion! Illusion is something which is already there — perhaps very deeply hidden — which one wants neither to see nor to accept. Imagination is pure and without lies. It is something which does indeed exist somewhere, but it has not as yet assumed any form. But there is always the possibility that imagination may become true or that it is already true. And it lies in our power to make it appear in a positive or in a disconnecting form. You must know that what people call 'negative' is a kind of behaviour resting on the illusion that everything is disconnected and that anything can occur without any connection with anything else.

Well, what I imagine determines my coming life. Before I have heard Papa's voice very clearly for the first time, and I have felt exactly what he wanted to say to me. This is the first time that he has spoken so directly to me[69]. I wonder if he has felt me as completely as I have felt him?

I am very happy, and would like to console you, Mama, about your stomach cramps. I am always with you, even unto the end of the world. I am embracing you with my little arms — will you feel it?

I would like to tell you so much more, but it is difficult to put it into words. Thus our conversation is not yet at an end. We will just lie quite still for a little while, just to feel each other. It will do much more for us than words.

It ends again with a deeper beginning. Manuji.[70]

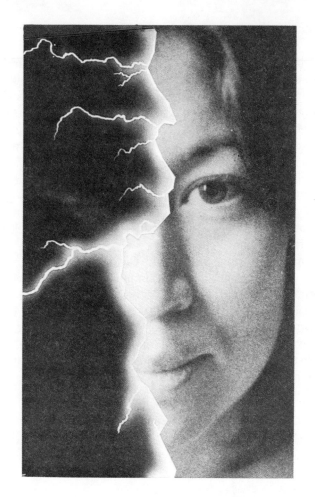

22.   *Not Only Loving Thoughts*

30th week of pregnancy, 22nd message.
Regional Women's Clinic, March 29th 1984.

Mama, why are you still playing with such heavy, gloomy thoughts[71] and allowing them to poison your body? Frequently you think: "Why must I suffer? Is there no end?" No, there is no end, because there is no suffering in this sense: there is only a struggling against something which you have yourself created.

Today we had not only loving thoughts and feelings. And you did not deny it. You honestly admitted your weakness in not being able to think of me always in a loving and joyous way.

It did not affect me, because during those thoughts you were somewhere else and not with me at all. Then, as soon as you were with me again and felt me, you were no longer able to have those heavy thoughts. How wonderful!

We have made the discovery together that being cross or dismissive happens only when we are inwardly not quite at one — when we have distanced ourselves from each other. I have discovered to my great surprise that you think sad thoughts only when you are not entirely in my heart. I am also no longer only in your heart — I felt that clearly today.

You asked outwardly what is to become of us, whether you would be able to carry me for my full term. You did not ask yourself what was happening just now. And that frightened you so much! The past seized hold of you again, and you let yourself be made defiant and fearful.

I can feel the questions you are asking of Life. Let us begin to question not Life, but ourselves. More and more carefully. I am often very hard and stern. I can be angry too, outwardly. You will see. A little of your inward resistance has transferred itself onto me. Earlier I wanted to be very hard and fierce with you. Did you feel it? You picked up a little of my fighting spirit and retained it, I know that. It helped you a lot.

In former lives we have been through much 'suffering' together, and we were 'drowned' more than once. But in this life you have not yet cleared up the question: does something happen because I fear it will? Or is my fear an anticipation of something already on the way? I feel your doubt, and I myself am beginning to meditate on it.

Can a baby in the womb meditate? That is what you are asking yourself at the moment. We will see later on, when we can speak with each other with our tongues.

I have a great many things which I want to accomplish. This moment, this situation, is familiar because we have already experienced it before. It's great to have a child. But can you have it really? Never. I hide a lot from you and the others in order not to be known and judged: your tummy protects me from that. Nevertheless, I had an impulse to come out of your tummy before, while I am still too small. An inner unrest and impatience coming from you was forcing me into it[73].

Also, you had a dream in which I said: "Mama, I want to come out". And you were strong enough to say to me: "You must stay inside for another hour". And I stayed there[72].

There are often dark, empty spots in your veins, which swallow up the stars of light in your blood. But we have enough stars to fill these holes[73].

Dear Mama, I am embracing you. The picture you carry of me in your heart makes me very happy. No matter what happens, I shall always be around you and the two of you.

I am wild and calm at the same time. Can you feel it? We must struggle: the very fact that we can shows us our power and freedom to stand above everything. Are you beginning to understand?

Now I want to speak just to you, alone again. This is meant just for the two of us. Don't write it down.

Do you love my inner wildness?

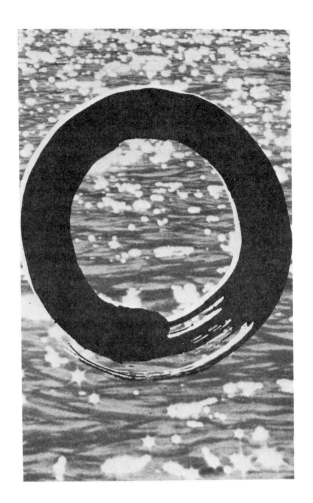

23. *Making a Circle of Power*

30th week of pregnancy, 23rd message.
Regional Women's Clinic, March 30th 1984.

Dearest Mama, again you see me inwardly before you — a picture of 'my' little baby — as you have seen it before. And now before you is the picture of me as a man[74].

113

We were disturbed — let us come together again[75]. Look into my eyes. Do not let us have any disturbing vibrations coming in to us.

I am embracing you. Let us make a circle of power. I can still feel your tension, which came when someone broke into our conversation. In reality, nothing can prevent us from talking to one another!

Well, so you used some technical apparatus[76] in order to lose your pretended uncertainty that I was a male! Please stop your so-called uncertainty in the face of negative vibrations!

I cannot say anything more to you now, because you are too taken up with yourself, and with overcoming intrusive vibrations.

I am with you. I will join you with my help. Let yourself be completely permeated by our force. Totally, absolutely, for ever.

Everyone is divine within. Never forget that.

Your baby is well. Let us become quite calm again together. Until the next time.

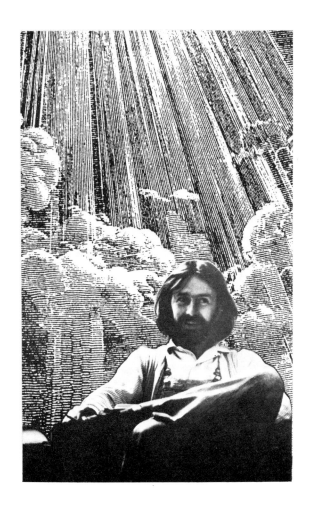

24. There is Such a Place as 'Heaven'

30th week of pregnancy, 24th message.
Regional Women's Clinic, March 31st 1984.

Dearest Papa, I was with you last night and saw you in your sleep[77]. So peaceful and deep, almost on your tummy, your head turned to the left. Your left foot was sticking out from under the blankets. I looked at you so tenderly, and loved you so much. You were sleeping deeply and dreaming. You were with me in 'heaven'.

Today you rang us up and telephoned me through Mama's tummy[78]. Your voice was much more lively and rested than last time. I got everything, and understood that you were speaking to me through an apparatus. It is wonderful for me, when you talk to me. You asked me a lot of questions. You always want to know so much! How am I to explain an experience to you? How have you forgotten that we have already been together in 'heaven', as you call it?

You were an old man at that time — because that is what you wanted to be. You had a white beard, brown skin, very bright greenish eyes and a young-looking face. Your beard was very long and you kept stroking it. And we were such good friends — very close, our friendship was very deep. Even then you wanted to learn such a lot from me. You keep asking me questions all the time and waiting for answers, which you then considered very carefully. Perhaps like now?

At that time you did not have any books. Perhaps it was then that your desire to record knowledge arose. I always tried to explain to you that you cannot 'hold on to knowledge'. Such a thing simply does not exist — not as you have always imagined it. No security — perpetual change is bound up with knowledge, with the knowledge that we humans have and must earn. True knowledge cannot be learnt, cannot be proven, cannot be stored up, cannot be won, stolen or copied, and can never be enquired into.

There is no such thing. It is just truth. Just being. Existence. It is very difficult for me to explain this.

Giving up knowledge is often the hardest thing for many 'seeking people'. It is not to be found on the outside, and not on the inside either. The great, deep 'being of knowledge' is endless and eternal. It cannot be expressed.

I have no knowledge. I am.

You have asked me about 'heaven'. Yes, it does exist. Like the earth and the other planets, like invisible and visible universes too. Heaven exists as a place. So does earth. But the earth, like heaven, also exists as an invisible experience.

The heaven you asked about, the visible 'physical' heaven is a free place. It is where one realises that one can do everything one feels the need to do. It exists independently of time and space. And you can go back there at any time, as soon as you have regained the remembrance in you, in your own inner heaven. Then you can travel quite easily to the outward heaven.

Your knowledge hinders you so much from travelling to that heaven. Even at moments when your gentle soul is quite ready, you let yourself be detained on earth by your reason and your knowledge.

And you cling to your so-called security. You already know well that one fine day you will be able to experience all you wish — when you have abandoned being bound to the earth, which at the moment is a necessity for you.

Up to now you have not doubted for a moment that you can travel in heaven. Can you not see that already, every second, you carry it inside you? And more often you withdraw into it. With me, with us, together or alone.

I will not tell you about the colours, the shapes, the circumstances and other such things about the external heaven. It wouldn't do you any good! You can find out about all that very well in your imagination. I know it, because we were there before. You do not need to ask about it, and you also do not need any confirmation.

But do you want a lot of other people to be told about it? Yes, that must be it. But I can only try with empty words to explain something which most people can grasp only with their reason, and which they might possibly believe. That is what most people seem to do. Some even blame themselves for their so-called flights of imagination. How sad for them that they have not yet learned to love life!

Would you like to make a journey with me without thoughts and questions? Without consideration and judgement? I am waiting for your answer in a dream.

You are so dear to me. I love everything about you. Everything, everything. It will be wonderful.

Mama, yesterday I was irritated by the cold apparatus and the sounds which penetrated deep into me[79]. It was like cold, sharp drops of water, which rained down on to my body and knocked each other off again. It was not equally hard on all parts of my body.

I felt your heartbeat becoming stronger and faster again. You were very shaken. It made you tremble. But you and Papa also had such deep, great joy. That relaxed my body, so that everything was well again. But I went on feeling the pricking and tingling for a long time, especially on the surface of my body. There was also a very gentle, pleasant voice in the room. I felt very much drawn to it[80]. You felt my impulse very strongly. You were almost surprised at your wanting to hug this voice.

I felt many dark figures creeping around in the building, but they never came near us.

Tonight I also visited the little babies[81]. I went right down amongst them. Many are still in the womb and a few are out. We felt each other — some are awake. The mothers understood nothing at all, but we babies understand each other very well. If one cries, another will often cry with it — but we do not all cry with it. Many of them are so alone that they are not properly aware of the other little ones — they are so clenched up.

Many babies who are already out tell those still inside about their births. Naturally, not in words. They share everything with each other. Do you think the mothers have any idea about that?

A tiny little girl is in the building. I like her very much. She is lying on a glass bed. I will frequently visit her in my dreams[82].

Neither of us is in a comfortable position. Let's stop. Papa is waiting so eagerly for our news. I send him everything . . . [83].

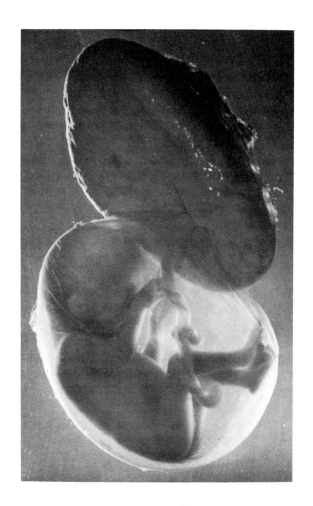

25. I'm Playing!

30th week of pregnancy, 25th message.
Regional Women's Clinic, April 1st 1984.

Mama, today I heard your mother on the telephone. Her voice is so timid and anxious. She is so attracted to me — she wants so much from me. She wants me — just as she wants you. She is waiting so much for me, but with great joy and in good heart.

Why is she so anxious? She has tensed the whole of her under-part, as though she had to hold everything together in order not to let anything out below. Her voice is like that of a little hare. All her hopes are fixed on us. We shall not be able to fulfil her wishes. I have an affectionate feeling for her, but I shall not let myself be affected by her vibrations.

I can feel how you accept her help, but inwardly you feel bad about it, because you are still dependent on her in this respect[84]. And that hurts you very, very much. That is the reason why the last little part of your self-confidence is still missing. It is only when you have managed to be independent of her in every respect that you will be sufficiently relaxed to regain your self-confidence completely. It will not be long now.

I am resting now in you, and am seeing 'heaven'. Oh! I see bright stars on a dark background and other joyful lights. And forms which float and hold hands with each other.

Tiny little beings are romping in the water beside me and playing with me. They are eating each other and then disgorging one another again — that is very amusing. One eats another and then spits it out at the back, whereupon the one spat out just swims away quite happily. There are other little beings in your tummy too — they are purifying the water all the time and shine like pearls of silvery red glass. Sometimes they become darker, sometimes lighter[85].

I feel stronger and stronger energy flowing upwards from the soles of my feet. My arms are becoming stronger and I am beginning to want to take hold of things, to seize them and carry them around.

I can contort my legs and also turn my head much more than I used to be able to do. My whole body plays in an ever more relaxed way, although there is getting to be less and less room.

Today I felt Lydia stroking me. It was strange, quite different from when you or Papa do it. It was so much further away. I felt her movements more than I felt her emotion, which inwardly would have touched me completely. And you gladly let her do it.

I like your way of talking to me, and I also sense when you find it difficult to speak to me only for the sake of writing down what I say — but, as you see, it all works, as I am still in your tummy!

I have begun to miss the walks. We must therefore go for a walk more often in imagination. That does just as well — it gives me almost as much 'fresh air' as if we really were in the woods.

This resting is very good for us though. And this lying down a lot is also very pleasant at the moment. I shall stay inside you a little longer. Your Manuji.

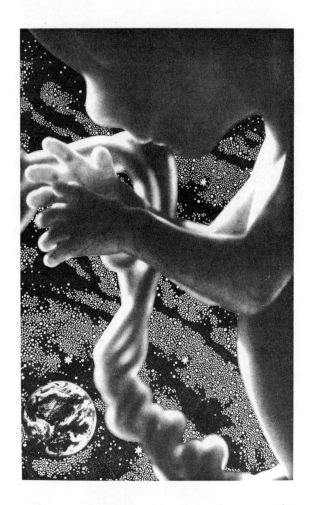

26. *Don't You Understand?*

30th week of pregnancy, 26th message.
Regional Women's Clinic, April 2nd 1984.

My dearest Mama, all deep wells within me are full of love and bliss when I feel you and am near you. I feel how you have become soft again.

The courage to keep silent. To stop doing something which, you told me, everyone does: talking about other people, thinking about them and judging them — without feeling and understanding. Stopping it? Do we have a secret? If the people round you cannot understand, will those who read our words understand?

Is it genuinely being silent if one speaks, yet keeps everything — or what has been said — locked up in one's heart? Is this to make you get strong? You are no longer afraid of showing it, yet you do not share with others around you what you know.

How deeply I feel for you!

Let us get rid of absolutely all doubt and let us not 'think' so much about everything we have said. It is unimportant. Over.

Each moment we are different. A different wave — and yet the same. Are you afraid of being a wave?

Mama, do you understand me? Now for the first time, I get the feeling that you cannot understand me completely. You are still a little distant.

I want to tell Lydia something. Very softly, secretly in her ear. But not here, in this book. No, not any more. I will tell it to her through you when she is near me.

She is so sad, so very, very sad. Why? Because she has hurt herself so much. Her accident was her own fault and that is breaking her heart. She will not believe there is any forgiveness deep in her heart. She cannot believe it. She blames herself for her 'deformity'. She struggles so much, reflecting outwardly what she refuses to accept inwardly. Is it from hardness?

I have a great deal more to say to her, but not here.

A little though, because it applies to many people . . .

After all, everyone in their own way creates their own fate. And she is still seeking hers. But she is seeking pain, deep pain. She feels it in her heart, and also seeks it outside. She seeks it! So she must find it — as long as she seeks it. But only so long as pain is sought — do you understand that?

The pain in a person's heart is there because it comes from the past. As long as pain is sought, it is easily found. Don't you understand? You seek pain in all sorts of different ways, whether it is stored up or in your imagination.

Must this be? I'm not the one who can answer that yet.

We also seek fortune and happiness, but we do not need to speak of it. It is everywhere! Like pain also? How is it that pain is seen in the same way, as if it were everywhere?

I am hidden inside you, deeply hidden. I already have a face, quite a definite one. It is only a little while until I am there, visible to your eyes.

But can you not see me already? Have you never asked yourselves: why can't I see something that is just behind a wall? Why must I go to the other side to see it?

It's just a wall between. And it is a reality which is behind it. I can check that — I need only to go behind the wall.

Dear Lydia, you are thinking of me, with sad and loving eyes. You want to be so brave. But why is it that tears come to your eyes whenever you think about being brave? I love you and will see your foot cured. Seeing is everything — how one sees something, and whether one sees it . . .

Manuji may now be nothing more than a very small baby. I would like to go to sleep, to rest and just be a baby. But it is so lovely talking to you that I can scarcely stop!

A circle of angels is standing around us protecting us with glowing torches, so that every word, every impulse, is allowed to be written down. You have the courage to start this, and the game must now be played to the end . . .

I feel that the link between my body and my talking with you is getting stronger. I can no longer move around inside you so easily, and neither can I reach you as easily — I am ever more strongly concentrated on myself, anchored in myself.

I feel your deep soul-wish to hear more from me, and to penetrate deeply into things, without its having to involve pain. Does it actually hurt?

Let's drop the distinction between hurting and allowing something to hurt — then we shall be alright. Is it so important if something hurts? It is just like any other experience.

At this moment. I do not want anything else but to lie inside you and hear the familiar music. We are flowing closer together, and our feelings and understanding are merging like many rivers flowing into the sea. Can you hear it murmur and rush?

Manuji loves you.

Should I not even mention the word 'loving' when you want to keep things silent?

I am smiling. And I am smiling at it. I am smiling at everything.

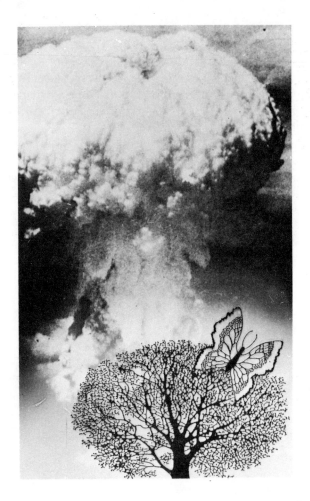

27.   *Life Cannot be Destroyed*

31st week of pregnancy, 27th message.
Regional Women's Clinic, April 3rd 1984.

When you give birth to something, you're letting it grow within you until it is mature enough to come out into the light.

Everything which grows within us will be born and is Life — it has Life within itself, if we permit it — as long as we do not interrupt the flow.

An embryo grows, and will, or should, be born. It has Life in itself. It is Life.

Who decides in what way Life will express itself? Who determines what Life is?

A child is conceived like an idea, like a thought. The wish, the power to let it grow, to gestate it, to bring it forth and let it make its way to completion is the very furtherance of Life.

Or: you can cut short the thought and suppress it. You can take away its energy, take away its power to grow and to reveal itself. You can break the buds off a tree . . . but it will get new ones! Life lives! And how it moves to reveal itself is left to it, itself.

All appearance is deceptive: Life cannot be destroyed . . .

You asked me this question before and used the word 'abortion'[86].

Each one of us hears his own life, and is responsible for his own life — as in small things, so in great ones.

Humans 'kill' animals. They try to kill Life. They only appear to do so. Everything is energy.

And what is behind it — everyone knows in themselves: just what you are at this moment, what you feel and wish.

I know only one sad story: humans believe they are able to kill themselves and so to kill Life.

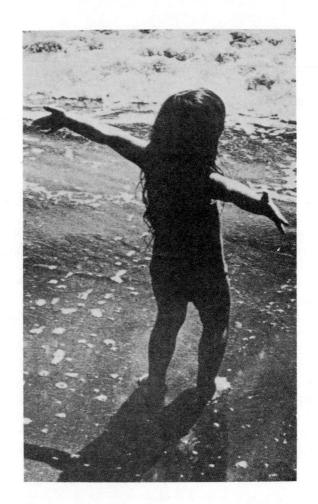

28.   Opening Oneself to 'God'

31st week of pregnancy, 28th message.
Regional Women's Clinic, 4th April 1984.

Mama, you are beginning to understand what *surrender* is. To surrender one's little will, to open oneself to 'God'.
Today you surrendered yourself completely to Papa[87]. And

Papa is our god. You very much resist writing this, but please do so. I, Manuji, am so happy to have been allowed to see you both in this situation today.

During the night your great pain before the 'breakthrough' began. Fear, as a separator, as a wall against Papa, against all and everything. Fear, this tightness, this pain which occurs when you are behind your defensive wall — and at the same time wanting to get out!

And how to open the wall? What is the magic word? You spoke that word to Papa today, and I experienced what was going on inside you — when you became more friendly to him. You dropped thinking of each other as a separate 'I' and 'you'.

How we all three suffered! And how it hurts when we all were behaving stiffly toward one another. It was an inner struggle for all three of us. I also felt how your fear, your locking yourself away from the birth of a new self, made you completely weak and helpless. But you succeeded. Papa succeeded to some extent too. We three succeeded — in loving one another without restriction.

How many lies we have told each other in the past in order not to surrender! Not to surrender our wills, our beings, and abilities to act.

Surrendering one's ability to act — that is something completely new for many people. To surrender one's ability completely to others, to Life.

Surrender means giving something up without asking anything in return, without expectation of reward.

I have also felt that sometimes you do not feel yourself quite ready for the great 'gift' that you feel me to be. And you believe that you could not give enough in exchange.

So many young people have had to learn the painful lesson of 'paying for love'. And they will have to unlearn it again.

I know about your fear of the medicines you have to swallow in order to keep me. The contradiction makes you very angry, deep inside you, because you know that you don't necessarily need them. But you're not yet sure of the alternatives. You feel your weakness in this direction, but you will learn a lot from it.

Medicines do me harm only when they remain inside me — if you do not relax and therefore fail to take care of eliminating them from your body and mine. Relaxation lets toxic agents leave the body. If the tension — often rooted in fear — lasts for some time, the medicines become stored up and begin to flood the body and form deposits, which become islands of decomposition or energy blocks — thus illness can arise.

Dear Mama, Manuji would like lots of kisses from you and would like to be stroked a lot!

I am beginning to wish something for myself — have you noted that? I want to hear your voice, and I so want you to talk gently and softly to me again. Especially when there is no one in the room and we are alone. We can be beautifully tender with each other.

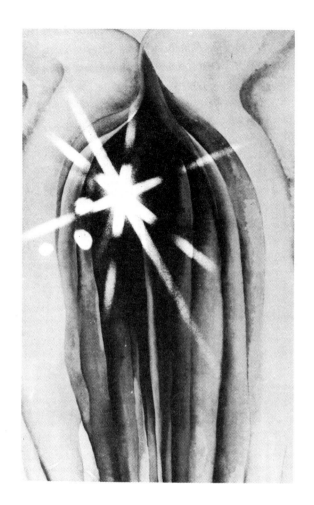

29. *Until We Soon Meet!*

31st week of pregnancy, 29th message.
Regional Women's Clinic, April 7th 1984.

Dear parents, please leave me in peace[88].
All my strength is now directed downwards, and I cannot
give you any more information.

It is too late. I have done enough to help you to understand. And I ask you now to help me and to give me peace.

Please accept my request. Until we meet again soon. Manuji.

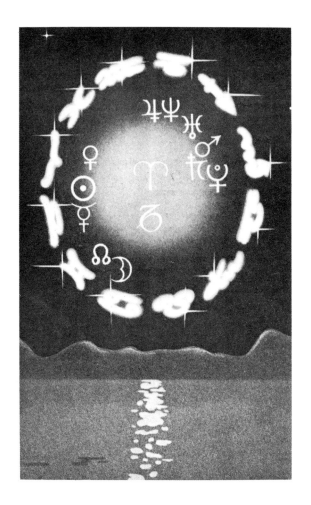

Seventeen Minutes Past Two at Night

Written by Mira

There they were again — my fears and uncertainties. I fought against them, as I had done before. If the coming experience was going to be positive for Manuji, I was going to have to subordinate my own feelings. It was a question of releasing my negative thoughts and opening myself up, no less.

My body was agitated. Hot and cold shudders went through me. I knew deep down I was entering a new and important phase in my life: it felt as if my body was beginning to weep. Ever stronger waves of pain were closing over me, and my throat was pulling tight.

My baby is coming too soon and there is nothing I can do about it. Why is he coming now? Why so early? Will Manuji be alright? How big and heavy will he be? Is he really a boy or a girl? Will he love me? I realised that I had not actually cleared up this last question — was I demanding love? Am I strong enough to love without expectation?

During all this, I realised I was expecting a lot. But this struggle to break ties did not last long. For two hours I tried in vain to put off the labour pains: when I realised this was impossible and ridiculous, I simply burst out in song! I was alone. René had not grasped yet that this was it — he had visited me in the afternoon, and seemed not to want to acknowledge what was happening. But subconsciously, he knew it was time.

I just lay there. For three weeks I had been a prisoner in this room. I could scarcely move, and was not allowed to do so — everything had to be done for me. My whole independence was therefore concentrated in my mind. My imagination was free to gather energy, which helped me go deeper into an inward state.

The question of whether or not the baby would live came to the foreground. I knew it would be small, and would probably be taken away from me, and I knew that the perineum would have to be cut. I could see everything clearly. Somehow I could feel exactly what was coming. The moment of decision had arrived. I shook myself and said: "Now you must take the plunge".

I took the step and fell tumbling into the depths. Immediately, the first really drastic contraction came — the pain decreased rapidly as soon as I went with it. I let the pains come over me with great wavelike movement. At each rush I said "Come". I spoke to the baby too, and loved him deeply. Then I had to let go: I must not keep Manuji any longer. In fact, I did not want to keep him any longer! I couldn't.

At this point, it came clear to me that I had been under extraordinary physical pressure and in great fear. I didn't fundamentally believe I was capable of having a child. Yet I had reached the point where it was happening anyway, regardless. Torment and despair washed over me. Then I felt a certainty that Manuji would live. Why, however, had I not had such faith or knowing before? I felt a deep resolve to demonstrate to myself that I could Do It — and that I would like to spend most of my labour alone. It struck me that this was the way I could rebuild my self-confidence from its foundations up.

I let myself sink deeper. Nurses and doctors came and went, but only one of them realised I was in my last stages of labour. The water had broken, and I had been given medicines in the morning — an injection of penicillin which I knew was not only unnecessary but harmful.

Memories of my last birthing arose. I wanted to depend on the experience of my first delivery, which had been easy, because I had gone into it so naively. I began to sing again. I repeated to myself that I mustn't become unconscious, and that I must welcome the pain — I was accustomed to going *with* pain. So hand in hand with it I went deeper into a strange land, knowing it would be difficult but beautiful there. I was cold and shivering. Then a new rush came.

In this state I rang René to say Manuji was coming tonight. At first he would not believe me, but he came by the last train. In the minutes following the telephone call, I learned how to free myself from my husband too — to allow him either to be here or not, as was best for him. Suddenly I realised that, having taken things into my own hands, I had the courage to stand behind my decisions wholeheartedly, and could let go of Manuji, let him come.

Half the night I lay in bed in this state, sometimes half-sleeping, but mostly awake. It was good to feel how strong I was with my pain, and how easily I was actually bearing it. I kept a positive feeling in me, and spoke to Manuji and stroked my tummy. Each time I stroked it, I wiped away more of the sadness and melancholia from my body.

René arrived, completely tired from dashing here, there and everywhere. He slept on the bed beside me. I experienced a feeling of great strength and solitude, as often before in my life. My baby and I, all alone — it was simultaneously beautiful and sad.

Early in the morning the rushes became severe and at regular ninety-second intervals. I hadn't had any bowel movements for two days and now I needed it! Blood! The birth was beginning. Now I would have to go up to the labour ward. After my previous two deliveries I knew exactly when the moment had arrived: a voice inside me clearly said "Now!".

I dressed and went quite normally up to the delivery room. A midwife was waiting for me, but she was rather hysterical. She could not equate my regular ninety-second rushes with the fact that the mouth of the womb had not dilated fully. She thought the rushes were cramps. What she said affected me slightly, but inwardly I was sure this was not a case of the cramps.

I was in a new state of consciousness: negative and restless vibrations had no effect. René was a very kind companion, and I noticed what a dear child he was — childlike in spirit rather than childish in behaviour. He sat beside me and held my hand. The midwife gave me a suppository — mainly to calm herself, not me — and left the room.

Then came the greatest waves of pain, and I was seized with the urge to run away. But I didn't: I stuck with it, knowing that by staying on the case I would succeed. I turned on the bed to make myself comfortable. Then came the first 'bearing down' rush. I uttered a small, shrill sound, whereupon the midwife rushed in, shocked that I had been right after all.

Manuji's head was visible, and the doctor quickly fetched the scissors. No more chance of free movement: I had to lie as they told me. That was strange, for I was sure I knew best and could do it. René protested to the midwife and helped me. After that, I was left in peace. However, when the perineum was cut I had to lie on my back. I can still see the long scissors hovering wickedly over my body.

I was conscious and wide awake like never before in my life. All my strength was directed into this work and I wanted clearly to accomplish it well. I pushed down, and gave myself over to the waves. I surrendered completely.

Then came the cut. I can still hear that crunching sound and feel the blood dripping between my legs. I felt the pain not in my body but in my mind.

And then, with a whoosh, Manuji was there. It was a wonderful experience that I had borne a child so easily. Actually I had done nothing but let go! That's what birthing is!

They placed him on my tummy. The look from his little eyes will stay with me all my life. It was the kind of deep and inner feeling I have only otherwise had with René. I stroked Manuji, this tiny little son of mine. How small he was! "He's very small, isn't he?" I said. "Yes, very small". René was thunderstruck. Everything had gone so fast for him — he hadn't expected things to land up like that!

Then our son was wrapped up, and we were allowed to ogle over him for a while before he had to go. I didn't want to be saddened by our parting. For the whole time I was strong and wanted only to transmit positive vibrations. I didn't know where they would be taking him, and could only hope all would be well — in the long run, it did work out well.

All that followed was terrible for me. I soon emerged from this lofty, conscious state and fell back into my fears and indecision. The cutting of the perineum had given me a shock, but I was, and am, continually nourished by my higher self, so I'll get rid of the shocked feeling bit by bit.

I thank Providence for this delivery and for sending us Manuji!

René writes . . .

When I arrived at the clinic, I was told that I could attend the birth only if I had attended the clinic's pre-natal preparation course for parents-to-be. I protested vigorously, and eventually a doctor said he might be able to do something to help. We had chosen this clinic because it was known to have a more progressive atmosphere than most.

After Mira's bad experiences during her first confinement — her husband had displayed a complete lack of interest — it was absolutely necessary for her to know I was at hand during these hours. It was really important to me to be present, too.

The evening before, when I was in Linz, Mira had rung saying that that night was going to be the night. This was by no means the first time! I wouldn't believe it. Partially, I had urged her earlier to put off the labour, if she could, since she was still premature, and also since the communications had not finished — in my estimation. However, by now I was more uncertain, and so I decided intuitively to catch the last train to Wels, where the clinic was.

I found Mira in good spirits listening to music on the headphones. After a few words of 'fatherly' encouragement, lying beside the two of them, I simply conked out with weariness, after the organisational exertions of the last few days. I was so tired that I wasn't much use to anyone! Too many things had been happening at once.

At about 10pm, Mira woke me up. It was only at this point that I fully recognised that Manuji was on his way. In order to be fit for a long night, I gently took my leave, rushed over to a cafe for a quick coffee. When I got back, psyched up and ready to go, Mira was singing again. I was pleasantly surprised, and proud of her. At midnight, she asked me to ring Caroline at home — Caroline was a midwife at the clinic who had resolved to be present at our birth, come what may. However, she misjudged the timing from my description of Mira's state, and arrived thirty minutes late!

I had made various preparations for the birth. None of them came to anything because everything happened so quickly!

I am told that a woman shows her true self and attitude to life in childbirth. If this is so, Mira's independent and unusual character was confirmed for sure. Her uncertainty was only on the surface. When it came to the crunch, she simply changed her role and started giving instructions to the medical staff. She decided the exact moment when the perineum should be cut (an essential thing in premature births).

After the final push, the baby gave a gentle cry. Not so loud and plaintive as I have seen in films. When Manuji lay on Mira's breast, he really seemed to be trying to talk. Not in words, but he demonstrated his dear little voice in a merry way. I was full of energy, wide awake and happy. I chuckled privately about the youngest author in the world coming to see the light.

During the afterbirth (the placenta was very small), our junior was bathed in the next room, measured (41cm) and weighed (1.56kg), and wrapped up to keep him warm. He was given to Mira again for a while, and then lay for ten minutes on a padded table beside an oxygen blower. Here I was able to speak to him alone. I explained that he would have to now go quickly by ambulance to the big Children's Hospital in Linz, and that he must now be strong, and that we shall be with him in our thoughts. I told him I found him beautiful, and that I would come to see him early in the morning. His wide-awake eyes showed me clearly he had understood it all. He then smiled, and I felt I was walking on air.

How Manuji felt during the journey in the ambulance he will perhaps tell one day!

After that, Mira's joy of motherhood was rather rudely interrupted by the nervous midwife. "She washed me as if I were a tin soldier" was Mira's description. The preparations for stitching the perineum followed. Mira consistently refused an anaesthetic in order to experience this part as well. Later, the doctor said that he had never before seen such a case of pain reduction without anaesthetic.

In the operating theatre, an amusing situation occurred. Mira was saying to the doctor and nurse that the midwife's nervousness arose from a high consumption of sugar (which was, incidentally, confirmed), when the said midwife entered behind Mira. The junior doctor who was stitching up Mira tried to indicate to Mira to be quiet, to no avail — so he bit her gently on the right big toe!

Caroline arrived soon after. She was not only surprised how quickly it had happened, but also how lively and alert Mira and I were in such a critical situation. She and Mira had a wonderful long talk lasting hours.

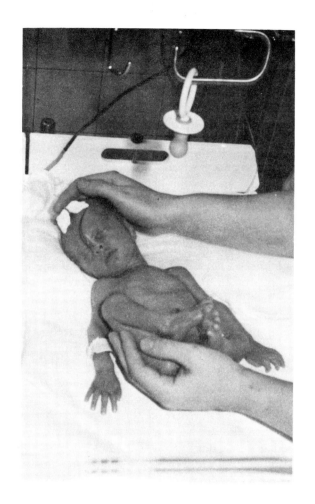

Five Weeks in a Little Glass Bed

Written by René

After a few hours' sleep, I arrived that same morning at the Children's Hospital. Since I was coming outside visiting hours, I had some difficulty getting in. After I had dressed in a white protective coat, pulled on plastic overshoes, and made my underarms sterile, I was finally allowed into the intensive care unit.

All sorts of machines were humming, fluorescent lights were flickering, and two young nurses were very busy, working away in a glass and metal environment. I was shown Manuel's little 'glass bed' by the window. He seemed to be the smallest of all the premature babies lying there. Above his forehead they had plastered on an infusion needle. I heard the oxygen intake tube hissing gently. Fully naked at an air temperature of 37°C, with a special humidifier, he lay on his back peacefully sleeping, his arms stretched above his head. His little feet were quite blue and bloodshot. I thought this must have happened during the birth — I learned later that it was because of the number of blood samples taken from his feet. Poor Manuji!

A friendly junior doctor came and gave me a short diagnosis. He said it would take two weeks before he could be sure Manuji would pull through. Otherwise, he said nothing special. I would be able to speak to the senior doctor another day.

Then they left me alone with Manuji. I found him outstandingly beautiful. How can the body of a premature baby look so mature? With his slender figure he was far more attractive than the chubby babies elsewhere in the room. He had a warmer colouring than the others too, and fine, unblemished skin. I reflected that it was not in vain that Mira has been so stringent about eating healthy food: the results were clear to see.

I opened the window of the incubator a little and began to whisper gently in his ear, telling him that I was there, that I loved him very much, and that I would, as far as possible, keep his connection with his Mama alive. After a time he smiled tenderly and slowly opened one eye. He was recognising me by my voice. When he was properly awake, he looked at me penetratingly and pulled a face as if he were going to cry — but he didn't cry after all. It seemed to me he was trying to indicate to me the treatment he had suffered, and his grief at being parted from us.

However, shortly afterwards, he radiated such a will to

survive that I could not be afraid for him. Cautiously I put my hand through the opening and touched him lovingly. He stretched his limbs in a way which was a joy to watch. I had my camera with me, so that I could at least take Mira some photos: when I began to snap him he adopted poses. I asked him to greet his Mama with a smile: after I had repeated the request several times, he made an attempt and then really did it. To this day, it seems to me to be a miracle that a premature baby could smile like that, just hours after birth.

I talked to him a lot more, and he listened attentively, staring at me with his little dark eyes and obviously enjoying the company and my voice. Then he became tired and fell asleep again, exhausted and content. Only then did I realise how hot it was in the intensive care ward — I was sweating profusely. Nevertheless, I stayed there until the end of visiting time.

Afterwards I reported everything to Mira on the phone. She had lots of questions, and was a lot calmer than I expected. Next morning I took the photos to Mira, and her eyes streamed with tears of joy.

On my second visit I found Manuji with a thin, transparent tube in his nose. Through this he had just received his first mother's milk (not his own mother's). Subsequently, I tried to spend as much time as possible with Manuji, and also visiting Mira. I was allowed to stroke Manuji only for a short time, in order not to let the incubator temperature fall, so later I tried letting the energy flow from my hands through the glass. Mira also, from her clinic bed, tried to be with him in her mind, and occasionally dreamed of (or with?) him.

The elderly staff-nurse on the intensive care ward became a problem though: she wanted to cut down my visiting times. I waved a leaflet at her which she had given me, which said "Your baby needs you!". Since I was persistent, I was given permission to come for extra time for the first week — but my doggedness had put me in her bad books.

I soon discovered why visiting times were restricted to the afternoons: in the mornings all the daily examinations and procedures were carried out — infusion needles were inserted, blood samples and X-rays taken, and other things. Every morning I saw a plumpish lady in white pricking the babies' heels and filling a small phial with their blood. Each baby screamed like a taunted pig. By the end of the week, I could hardly bear to watch the process. Manuel always calmed down afterwards, but I was moved to question the doctor how necessary this pricking really was.

I was referred to the head doctor, whom I had understood to be a very kind man, but he gave me an entirely different impression: he hardly let me say a word and would not look me in the eye, reciting the official jargon and then wanting to go. To my question about blood samples he retorted: "This is not a research laboratory!". I didn't understand the relevance of his answer, or his nervous behaviour until I found out later about a recent media scandal, in which a Viennese children's doctor had been carrying out scientific experiments without parents' knowledge. This doctor was apparently acquitted by the court, but the issue was a touchy one at the time. I didn't tell Mira about the matter.

Mira writes . . .

Since Manuji was no longer inside or with me, I lunged into a downswing, more frightful than the previous weeks. I was heart-broken at not being able to be with him. I could not sleep, because he wasn't there. I was also regularly disturbed by all the bed-making, the examinations, the various visits, and a tormenting feeling of mental pain which I couldn't release. Subjectively, it was like a torture session. My veins were pricked to pieces by continual injections. Yet, strangely, in another part of myself I was in a euphoric state.

My physical recovery was rapid, even though I was missing out on the important post-natal aspect of intimacy with my child. I wanted to be let out as soon as possible, and was soon up and about. The milk in my breasts came quickly too. René took bottles to Linz every day, and returned with news of how the baby was: for a week he acted as a courier between us. Apparently, Manuji had, after a few days, stopped needing many of the infusions and medications a premature baby usually has, and was classed as being very healthy. I also had the feeling I did not need the clinic any longer.

After five days, I was able to persuade the head doctor to let me go at last. In Linz, mercifully, a friend placed an unused room in her flat at our disposal. But it was dark, and René and I, after months of hardship, were both close to collapse. We would just have to survive thankfully with what we had.

Here are some entries from my diary.

At last I can see Manuji! When I entered the room in the intensive care unit, I was almost drowning inwardly in my tears. Manuji had lost a lot of weight and was alarmingly thin. But at the same time I felt joy that the connection between us was intact and nothing could destroy it. Perhaps it had even been strengthened by the hardship and separation we had gone through.

I stroked my little son. He opened his eyes and smiled. He has precisely those big, dark, wide-awake eyes which I had already seen in my meditations and dreams. It's taking me some time to accept how tiny and helpless he is in that glass box. I am still very weak, and sometimes I collapse in my chair.

Today, René played our alpha-music to Manuji, without the nurses seeing. He put a tiny loudspeaker under Manuel's padding and led the cable through his sleeve to the tape recorder hidden in his pocket. Manuji listened attentively, and certainly remembered the music.

On Manuji's medical record board it says 'Nothing special. Vital'. They judge him to be lively! Every two hours, a transparent, flexible tube is inserted into his nose, and he is fed milk through it. Suddenly, he is no longer hungry. I am convinced he would manage quite well at my nipple, for he sucks my finger already. When no one is in the room, I train him at sucking. But I may not give him my breast until he has reached a certain weight. Orders are orders. I hope all this has not done Manuji irreparable harm.

The whole business of expressing milk from my breasts by special hand pump takes an hour each time, six times a day. Travelling to Manuji takes an hour, and the same time back. This scarcely leaves me time for looking after myself, cooking food and other things.

Apart from a slight rash, Manuji is doing well, gaining weight, and has no complications. The doctors are duly surprised! I attribute the skin rash to the penicillin injections I had before he was born. The doctor denied any possible connection. An older nurse, however, overhearing the conversation, later said that she had had the same thing happening with her. She also said "Never talk to a doctor about medicines!". I shall remember that.

Today something wonderful happened. When I returned from visiting Manuji, I noticed that my hands were highly charged with energy. I had stroked Manuji for a long time and irradiated him, and I felt my healing abilities returning. When I sat down to meditate shortly afterwards, I could feel Manuji's 'etheric body' as strongly as when he had been there in the flesh. I was blissfully happy, and cradled him imaginally in my arms. Now I know that my inner approaches to him have been successful, and this gives me the strength to cope with the physical separation, and to make room for joy at Manuji's being alive.

René is away a lot, seeking to organise our future life. He might have found us a place to live, but that awaits confirmation... It ended up not working out.

In the morning I arrived at the hospital and could not find Manuji. He had been moved to the new-born babies department. He now lies in a warm cot, and is free of the incubator. For the first time, I could embrace his body and feel him properly. I am the happiest mother in the world! Even in such a strange situation.

Manuji gets his milk exactly to the minute and always in the same quantity. Today I was allowed to bottle-feed him. He did not want to feed at the breast — it was said it was too tiring for him, which I thought to be a strange notion. I'm sure he'll soon take to it. My milk is increasing all the time.

Most of the information the doctors give about all this is not very constructive. One laughed at us because we visit Manuji so often and for so long. I find it easier to leave Manuji today, since he obviously notices I am with him in his thoughts. Soon he will be heavy enough to be allowed home. Although our hopes of finding a home have again been dashed, I feel confident we'll soon have one to go to.

One of the nurses said today "Emanuel is awake a lot. He scarcely cries, and looks around with his big eyes, while most of the children are sleeping most of the time. Probably he's thinking to himself 'sleeping is too dull for me!'".

Another nurse has noticed Manuji's style. She said that, as far back in her working life as she could remember, she had never looked after such a baby. Manuji was amazingly contented, but what surprised her most was the way he observed everything alertly, so much like an adult. When he looked at her with his wide-open eyes, she sometimes felt 'quite strange'. Most babies still seem to have a vacant look. Just hours after entering the world, he had been smiling and fully engaged with things.

One afternoon I found Manuji wanting to suck, and I asked if I could bottle-feed him. He guzzled it all down like a little tiger, though it was not as tiring for him as the staff had anticipated. In the corridor you can hear babies crying all the time — I have to pull myself together so as not to cry with them. They instruct us not to take the little ones out of bed too much, since it tires them — but what about the crying?

Today, my baby fed from the breast for the first time, sooner than the doctor had expected. I am sure it was because of the practice I had given him with my finger. Now he is sleeping peacefully. I love him so much. The neighbouring babies are crying a lot — I don't blame them, for if an entirely unknown vibration replaces that of their mother, they have every right to feel upset.

Despite living in temporary quarters and dire straits, I am now feeling happier than I have in all of the recent years of my life. Perhaps it comes from the feeling of having done my duty to the best of my ability. I'm not meditating regularly, but when I do, I draw a lot of strength from it. Because my meditation is not so regular, its effect is all the more outstanding.

Manuji's baby neighbour, Claudia, had gone the full term, but was being kept two months in hospital. Apparently something is wrong with her heart, and up to now she has not been able to suck or swallow. Yesterday I could not bear seeing her plight any longer. When she finally fell asleep, I made contact with her higher self and spoke quite sharply to her. I assured her that she could drink, and she just had to try with all her might. I concentrated on persuading her. Lo and behold, today the nurse exclaimed joyfully that Claudia had taken to the teat.

They keep asking me when I am going to have my child vaccinated. I replied that we were thinking it over — though, between us, we will not allow it. The staff simply cannot understand that one can have a different opinion about it. We did think of giving them an Anthroposophical (a philosophy developed by Rudolf Steiner) leaflet about vaccination, but decided against it.

In German, the word for 'hospital' is 'Krankenhaus', sick-house: if only doctors understood the psychology of medicine better, they would call it a 'recovery house'. Just as fevers in a body already indicate a process of healing, so it is with other illnesses — they are eruptions of the effects of previous imbalances of body and mind, in which the body is confronting and repairing itself. That people do not recognise this means they are never fully healed.

Manuel is given sugared vitamins every day in his food. Today he has a watery, discharging eye. I believe this is a symptom of bodily rejection of the vitamin supplement. He now weighs 2280g.

The ward is mad. All around, children are screaming and howling, and people are coming in and out all the time. Sometimes I get the feeling I can see too much, and am over-sensitive. Most of the babies are visited but seldom: I do a round, and give a little of myself to them too. The factories outside the hospital are sending out a terrible stink today. It amazes me that a hospital is located adjacent to them.

I asked one of the doctors when I could take Manuji home. First he must drink properly for a few days longer, was the reply. Within a week, Manuji had mastered everything. He would be able to come home the day after tomorrow. I found all that difficult to grasp.

Six weeks have gone by, and I told Manuji "Soon you will come home — I've got a lovely little basket ready for you". He laughed all over his face. I could spend all my time chattering to him. While I am writing, I'm holding his little left hand. Now he is going to sleep.

Manuji's stay in hospital, two months in all, was a sad experience for René and myself. The staff had said some really crazy things to us: that we were visiting him so often only out of egotism, that we should stop stroking him so much (after all, a baby isn't stroked in the womb, is it?). To them, a premature baby is in a sense not fully born: did we honestly believe it was a complete human being? Then there was the ongoing struggle over visiting hours: it was scandalous to have to beg for access to one's own child! Then, during the last week, a large splinter of glass was found in the bottle from which we had been feeding Manuji.

As you might imagine, the stress we had to deal with from the management was quite unbearable. René was continually having to calm me down. The head nurse could not stand us, and she stirred up the head doctor with prejudices against us. When, on handing over the baby on our departure, he had asked if we were satisfied, René replied "90 percent", to which the doctor reacted in a remarkably emotional manner. "You will have a lot more trouble with that child", he said, "and you're demanding too much from that baby."

For weeks on end, Emanuel had accepted everything quietly and bravely. It seemed that nothing could disturb his composure. For us, though, it took several days to awaken from this nightmare and find our equilibrium again. This was underlined by an article we read about Third World techniques in childbirth: premature babies are simply wrapped up and tied to their mother's body, where they receive warmth and breast-feeding. This place of security is maintained day and night, and mothers and babies are thus able to leave hospital within one week — not seven, as we had to do. Austria has sophisticated medical technology and also, apparently, a surplus of doctors, but in spite of this it has one of the highest infant mortality rates in Europe! Something's not quite right there!

We had discovered a lot of things not to be right. But we were thankful for all that we had received. Manuji was with us.

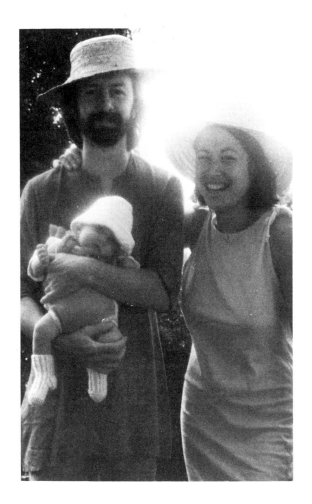

In the Driving Mirror

Written by René

When Junior was finally released from the hospital —
weighing 2.43kg — our odyssey was by no means over. In
spite of all my endeavours, I was not able to offer my wife and
son an acceptable home — which certainly hit my self-respect as

a father and man. We didn't want to ask Manuji to accept the dark boxroom in our friend's house either. We were in luck, though: a family offered us their flat in town, which they were not using at that time. However, we stayed but a few days. We wanted to leave Linz as soon as possible!

At that time, my father had been in hospital for some weeks with cancer. As a result, my mother secretly gave us permission to use their summer house for a short time. So, while Mira stayed with Lydia, I quickly renovated one room, in order to make ready our seventh provisional home.

My father never saw Emanuel. I could only show him a few photos of his fourth grandchild while he was on his sick bed. He let them drop out of his hand — he was conscious only for short times. He wasn't open to spiritual healing, so we couldn't do anything for him. For a long time he had not been on good terms with any of his sons, and this was reciprocated. Our lifestyles were too unconventional for him. When our father's end came, it had been so quick that none of us had been able to make our peace with him. On the day of his departure, two months after Manuji's birth, I was permitted to be with him, and prepare for his journey to the other world. I helped him with all my strength to turn his death-struggle into a peaceful release. He finally died with a smile on his lips. To be able to do this with him was a release for me. To experience the river of life flowing through the generations in such a concentrated way was very uplifting for me, a feeling of being at home in the cosmos. I believe now that my father's discontentment with me is ended.

From early summer on, we lived temporarily in the damp bungalow. Manuel slept in his Moses basket, but when going to sleep he likes to lie on my or Mira's tummy and let himself be rocked to sleep by the motions of breathing. He was still so tiny that we would bathe him in a soup pot.

At four months, Manuji caught a bad cough — probably from his Granny. Premature babies are very susceptible as far as breathing goes. In the night he was burning with fever, and

Mira panicked. We took him to a children's doctor, who thought he was on the verge of pneumonia, and went on to prescribe antibiotics. If Manuji was not better in two days, we would have to take him to hospital. He looked at us suspiciously, seeing that Manuji had been premature, and we had given him no vaccinations.

Babies have their specific illnesses in order to build up their immune systems, to become more resistant. We reckoned we would spoil his chances by giving him antibiotics, which kill everything indiscriminately. Confronted with Manuji's fever, Mira's fears and my own sense of helplessness, I came up with the idea that Mira should meditate and ask her dead teacher, Zeané Lao Shin, for advice.

Mira wasn't confident about this, but agreed to try. She withdrew to a nearby wood, where my brothers had laid out an Indian Medicine Wheel — a ritual circle marked out with stones in a definite pattern. She sat down with pencil and paper by one of the trees there, and went into meditation. With tears in her eyes, she begged her master to help with his wisdom. About thirty minutes later she heard his voice, and wrote it down:

You must remain open. Do not shut yourself up. Keep your eyes open and maintain peace in your heart. Look at great Nature and see what is done to her! Yet she remains silent and patient.

Be a rock. You know the Way, so follow it without hesitation. You will receive an indication of something you have not yet mastered. Remain open. Shutting yourself up hurts and separates. Do not despair. Yes, give it to him (the antibiotic remedy). You will see. It will certainly make him ill. But give it to him. You must give it to him, for otherwise he has no chance at all. He is strong, but he may die, so give it to him. If he dies in spite of it, at least you have given it to him.

He is strong, but his body is weakened because he is very 'Yin': you will not be a able to balance this for a long time. You must be very much on the alert, because up to his thirteenth year he may easily die. But if he dies, it does not matter. He will come again — have no fear about that!

Do not be so anxious. Your debt has already been paid. Now you are, so to speak, experiencing atonement: it will make you strong if you remain calm and have faith. Otherwise you will not make progress!

It will not be very bad. I am there if it becomes really bad. I am going now. You have heard my advice.

The message shocked us. For some hours we were incapable of making a decision, until a flash came to us, showing what Zeané had really meant. He had behaved with us in the way he often had done with his pupils. He was entering into our imaginary anticipations, addressing our fears so directly that we had no option but to wake up! A master of macrobiotics is telling us to use antibiotics: what a contradiction, yet how sensible!

Finally, we didn't submit Manuji to medicine, doctor or hospital. We took an old household remedy: onion poultices on the chest for a few days, radiating healing energy through Mira. He coughed a little more but was soon well again. The whole worry was over.

We lived almost six months at the cramped little summer house. In the autumn, Mira had another mediumistic contact, marginally connected with the baby. She had not been very well, feeling cramped living in but one room. Other people were using the other rooms during the day. She was sitting at the table, lost in thought, looking out of the window at the wood opposite.

Mira writes . . .

I was not thinking about anything, just vaguely looking out. Then I discovered a giant face, formed by the shadows of the treetops. I looked away, and then back, and it was still there. I said to René "I can feel a contact . . . ". He fetched a pen and paper. I looked again at the face in the wood and wrote blindly on the paper. René then reconstructed the message from my scrawl. This is a shortened version:

All love. All love. Tell them all love from me and my friends. We are the spirits of the wood and we guard and protect all beings who come to us, who come in us. We hear their speech.

I am very old and wise, as you would say. My face is constantly changing, like the hours of time. I hear it rustling all the time, for the speech of our hearts is music. I — we — listen for your voices and have heard your cry for help. We hear your singing and your crying. Your music finds an echo in our hearts. Be comforted, for you have called us and we will help you. We will protect your baby too . . . (Here there was an interruption). . . . No matter how much noise, we can always speak to you. We are awaiting your silent prayer and obey every invitation to dance. We love you and belong to you . . .

In this way I re-established contact with the elementals I had lost my links with in early youth. The last such contact I had had was with a birch tree.

René writes . . .

Mira's extreme sensitivity was demonstrated in another incident during the summer. Manuji had developed a rash, and so Mira took some propolis (bee glue) tablets, since they have a natural healing power, and we reckoned it would pass through Mira's milk. A few hours later Mira complained of a continual buzzing inside her. Shortly afterwards, a picture of a tree-stump in a wood, with a swarm of bees on it, came into her mind, and we laughed as we realised the connection.

Just before the winter of 1984-85 we had success at last with accommodation. In Attersee, in the heart of the Salzkammergut, we found — largely by 'chance' — a whole house, newly built and fulfilling all our wishes. Manuji's advice on his 21st message, to visualise a house with mountains near it, has thus been more or less fulfilled.

Mira writes . . .

Both René and I feel certain that Manuji takes in everything which goes on around him, and has done so ever since birth. He has an intelligent, piercing look which betrays his inner strength and calm. We are learning a lot from associating with him!

Apart from the time at the hospital, Manuji has never had a bottle. Up to when his first teeth appeared, my milk sufficed, delivered without packaging. I allowed him to suck at the breast whenever he wanted, and we never had any problems with him. He does not even suck his finger. His first solid food was creamed brown rice. It is very amusing to see Manuji's little fingers playing with single grains of rice. He has never had ready-cooked baby foods.

Many people say you have to sacrifice yourself when a baby comes. We have experienced the opposite. Emanuel directly touches our inner selves. Through him we are becoming more creative, and are clarifying what is important for us. It's wonderful to see him growing day by day. Many of our friends have already opened their hearts to Manuji, and his messages. This has deepened our relationship with them. It has been good to circulate Manuji's messages, and receive feedback.

Our little son is beginning to make pre-words with his mouth — *Huh, Mama, bapabapa, ungah* are his favourites at the moment. He sings along with tunes on the radio, and with the meditation music we play him, and bangs away happily on the keys of his toy piano. Then he quietens down and watches the birds through the glass door of the terrace.

Latterly, Manuel has been studying new people carefully before deciding whether or not to smile. At home with us he laughs a lot, and cries only when he has a serious problem. Truly he has a friendly disposition.

A few days ago we had a visit from a woman in an advanced

state of pregnancy. I stroked her tummy and spoke out loud to the embryo, and sent her baby loving rays of energy through my hands. The mother confessed to us that she had never before in her pregnancy felt such strong, direct reactions from her baby.

Through Manuji I have become strong. In this pregnancy, I was so earnest and my experiences were so deep that I found the strength for lasting inner change. In spite of our separation after birth, I have felt an unbroken joy in his presence, ever since conception. Now we both have a deeper understanding of the biblical saying: "Except ye become as little children, you shall not enter the kingdom of heaven".

I wish to thank all of our friends, relatives and acquaintances, especially the spirit-helpers from the other side, without whose support the book would not have been possible. I am happy about the book: it has kept our experiences with Manuji so much alive. I hope our accompanying text will be of as much value as the communications, in putting everything into the picture.

When a child arrives, it wants only to express love. It cannot understand rejection of love. It loses its confidence, and the courage to demonstrate its love. Bad upbringing produces a society such as our own. It is, bluntly put, the duty of all of us to awaken to the here-and-now, and help the children of the future be happy, even while in the womb, so that they can take on a new quality of life.

The question arises about why Manuji's messages ended when he was born. René could not see the reason for this, however much he turned it over in his mind. The upshot was, he said that the best thing was to try to establish contact on our side. I then tried meditating beside the sleeping baby and tuning in to him. Almost immediately, Emanuel woke up and looked at me in astonishment. René would not be content with this, and spoke to the baby about his problem. A few days later, when René was away, I tried again. I meditated in the bedroom on the first floor, and Manuji was lying on the sofa in the living room below. For a long time, nothing happened, and I was about to give up, when something came . . .

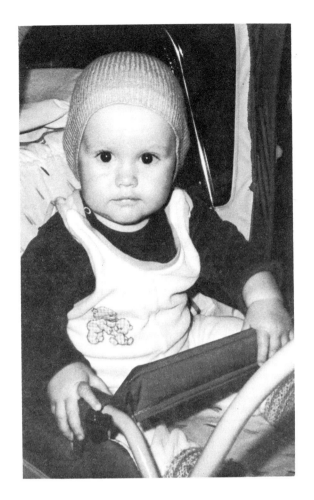

30. Mummy, Listen . . .

11 months after birth, last message.
Attersee, March 15th 1985.

M ummy, listen, please don't write anything more about me in the book. Mummy, Manuji is unhappy if you write something else in the book.

We parents took a middle course between Emanuel's wishes and the expectations of our readers, by publishing this message, but only bits of it.

Neither do we want René to write any more in the book, in any way which is connected with little Manuji. We are his protectors and beg you now to leave him in peace with the book. He has fulfilled his task and must now live his babyhood undisturbed. So far he is well . . .

He is very open and you must protect him from false projections which might affect his personality if his present being should be publicised in an unbecoming way. Please trust your inward advice and leave Manuji in peace to be an innocent, unknown being in his present life. He has earned the right to it, and he owes nothing to anyone.

He can now decide for himself what he would like to do with his life. His activities depend entirely on his own natural decision-making. And for now that is to be silent and to remain unrecognised.

The contact which you parents have with him is your own gift and is not intended for the masses. Every mother must deal with her child in her own way. And if she has understood Manuji's messages, she will now know what is to be done after the birth of her child.

Take care that he is not made into an idol, but rather is taken as an example toward which everyone can strive . . .

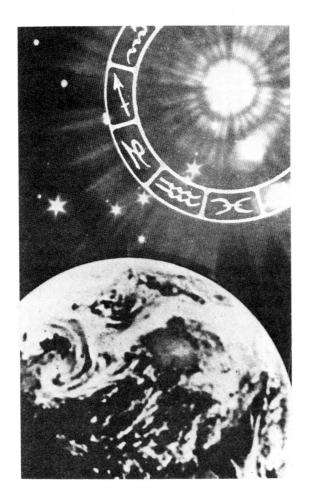

Epilogue

We feel that the world is entering a new era, and that the old order is gradually declining. Our personal sphere of activity is oriented toward such a future, and new areas of activity have opened up. We shall continue to spread Manuji's message as widely as possible, initially through further transmissions, and also through a film we are currently working on (1991). During the last few years, dozens of souls in the process of incarnating have communicated, through Mira, with their parents-to-be, which might appear as a book which serves as a sequel to this one.

In order to provide a happier time in the womb, and a happier childhood for as many little people as possible, Mira has a very special project close to her heart. This is to set up 'embryo-schools', similar to those which once existed in China. These would be a combination of seminar and recreation centres for pregnant women, in which, in harmonious surroundings, they would be given the opportunity to find keys to complete motherhood. Mira is very committed to this.

It is true that the potential of a people receives its stamp in the womb of its mothers. During procreation, the desires, thoughts and feelings of both parents play an important part. The coming together of a man and a woman to procreate is, ideally, a very loving act, one which lays the foundation stone for a temple of the flesh, into which a soul may enter. At the moment of birth, the parents make a pact with the soul which is hoping to incarnate — though often they do without knowing it. It is no secret in esoteric circles that the principle of affinity of vibrations also applies, in accordance with which the future child and its parents feel drawn towards each other.

It is probably not until pregnancy is well under way that the consciousness of the incarnating being slowly moves into the subconscious. Such processes vary from one individual to another, and naturally karmic backgrounds play an important role. After fertilisation, there will be a stage in which the spiritual attitudes of either the mother or the child will be established as the dominant one. In every case, however, the mother's inclinations towards beauty, harmony and health will have a positive effect on the developing child.

Thus, pre-natal education plays an important part in the new era. Yet, from the very beginning, a child belongs to itself, and has its own plan to realise. A caring mother, simply by being herself, will provide her embryo-foetus with a loving and considerate education. By contrast with current practice this will help the incarnating being to maintain contact with its own self. Then, as a rule, with the child's first breath, the soul which has entered will unite with the little physical being, and at the same time, the subtle energies present overall at that moment will play its part in the awakening aura which has just been set free. Asians, who are generally more conscious of such matters, regard little children (up to about the age of three) who have not yet developed the power to distinguish between good and bad, as God-like creatures.

As soon as the mothers of the world become more conscious of their task and of their inner power, our planet will increasingly become peopled with splendid beings. Thanks to the power granted by nature to women and accepted by them, the people of the future will all one day be healthy, warm-hearted and clear-thinking. Spiritual healing and psychic communication with higher intelligences will probably become commonplace. Toward such an end, we are preparing further material on our trance experiences, derived from several hundred hours of contacts recorded in writing and on tape. We no longer wish to keep this to ourselves, but we must ask our readers for patience, for it will take some years before everything is ready.

We wish to give a brief account of what has been — and continues to be — our most important contact. This inner dialogue began in 1985 when we were worried about an infection which Mira picked up. Since we had neither car nor telephone at the time, and there was no homoeopathic practitioner in our area, we had to face the problem on our own, since we refuse — except for diagnosis — to have anything to do with a medical practice which deals solely with *symptoms*. The only solution to our problem lay with mediumship. Our first attempt was an astonishing success, with a new and promising contact.

When she became ill, I advised Mira — though I had no definite idea what would happen — to try and summon a wise physician from the 'other side'. It took her ten minutes to become attuned, and then she transmitted, in a flood of words, an extensive and comprehensive answer to our questioning. The being speaking through Mira finally introduced himself, in reply to my insistent questioning, as Carl Gustav Jung (no less). We would not have wanted to mention his name here had the message not been one of such high quality, and if so many Jungian analysts had not confirmed that it was at the level of Jung's work. The content of the message was too far-reaching to be appropriate to present here, but we do want to reproduce a few aspects of it.

After we had received the homoeopathic medical advice we were seeking, I took the opportunity to ask Herr Jung if he knew the reason for Manuel being born so early. Until then, we had not been able to find a satisfactory answer. Was it that Mira's muscles were too weak? Was it her fear of premature birth? Or was it the stressful situation into which we had manoeuvred ourselves?

'Dr Jung' informed us in his detailed analysis that mainly for psychic reasons, there had been a misdirected flow of physical energy which prevented the baby from growing any more. In addition to a theoretical discourse on the latest discoveries of his research group 'on the other side', whose spokesman he was, we also received a surprising offer from the renowned psychologist which we gratefully accepted. "*We hereby express our desire, through this medium, to establish contact with those who have an inner longing to learn more about the whole process of their psychic energies, in order that we may together be able to serve mankind. By means of examples, we want to spread the knowledge which has reached us at a higher stage of wisdom. We achieved it by long experiment, testing, investigation and experience, and through the holy nature of our intention.*"

I, Carl Gustav Jung, am a disciple of knowledge and intuition and a great lover of the psyche, which is a gift of the unconscious to mankind. We should not harm it, and we should have no fear of the way in which it manifests, though this may often appear inscrutable to us. Shall we dare to penetrate into the very depths of our soul, which is at the heart of our psyche?'

Thus a new project fell into our lap, and has been in operation now for six years. Eight books have already resulted from this teamwork, four of which have already been published (in German).

Toward the end of my first conversation with 'Carl Gustav', which lasted for almost an hour, I introduced into this dialogue the subject of this baby book.

Yes, we have heard about it and we are pleased. He is a very sensitive little fellow, but he is nevertheless sufficiently steadfast to prevent confusion in his energy system.

We can confirm this statement. Manuel's inner calm soon became evident enough, though it took longer for his ram-like nature to manifest itself in the desire, metaphorically speaking, to batter his head against a wall.

Here is a last story about Manuji which is important for us. While he was still preparing himself to be born, Mira received a little chestnut tree as a present from a friend. She soon fell in love with the little plant, and irradiated it with tender loving care as if it were her own child. Since she was rearing this little tree in parallel with her pregnancy with Manuel, she attached a special importance to it. Soon the tree acquired a second stem, growing out of the earth. Surely, we thought to ourselves, this is an omen that Manuel is to have a little sister.

Six years ago we wrote down this conjecture, and today our little daughter Samantha is more than two years old. What is more, she came into the world in the same clinic as Manu, in an unusual case of full-term 'home-birth-in-hospital'. That is to say, she was delivered by me, single-handed, since there was neither doctor nor midwife in the ward at the critical time. A surprise at the birth had indeed been announced through the mediumship of a guardian spirit, but we had not dreamt of such an unusual delivery!

The urgent question which naturally arose was whether an intensive pre-natal mental contact had taken place with her, as it had done with Manuji. We had to answer in the negative. It is true that we had already sensed our daughter very strongly at the time her soul entered, but unlike Manuji she had not chosen to take a task upon herself. This she very quickly intimated. In direct contrast to her brother, whenever Mira tried to speak to her she would say something like "*Mummy, you are tired. Why don't you lie down and sleep?*"

There was, however, one long and very personal contact, but at our daughter's wish, we are not publishing this. On the other hand, Mira did have a number of meetings with Samantha in her dreams. For a time it was rather a worry to us that our second child felt no need to deliver any special message to us, but since her birth we have come to understand this. She shows us very clearly what a wonderfully self-determining person she is. She is proud of her elder brother and is simply the perfect completion of our family.

Finally, we would like to grant the wish expressed in many of our German readers' letters, to tell a little about Manuji's life. After the last proper message, there were a few more contacts with his higher self, but these were not intended for publication. Mira meditated beside him and became attuned to his spirit while he was sleeping in his cot. The very last contact of this kind took place during the hernia operation which he had to undergo when he was two, and which he came through with flying colours. He had trouble with his lungs too, as Mira's teacher had foretold, but he is now well over the worst.

He has a very clear memory of his glass bed, the incubator, because the tube through which he was fed with milk apparently scratched his throat. That he had so ably worked his way through the dramatic days following his birth was shown during a joint meditation involving Manuji and us, when he was about three. On this occasion he slipped into a spontaneous, non-verbal regression, back to the time of his first days on earth. Quite perceptibly, before our eyes, his face suddenly took on the features of the first days of his life, and he emerged from this state as though he had been healed of a trauma.

He has an enormous talent for drawing, and we already have several boxes of little masterpieces. At the moment, dinosaurs and pirates are his favourite fantasies. Now and then he still likes to have something read to him from his book, since he has already forgotten some of its messages. Then he slips under the blanket with Mira and wants to play at 'being baby in her tummy', waiting to be born. When he does this, he always explains that he only wanted to come out of her tummy for a moment to see what it looked like outside, and he didn't know that once you were born you couldn't go back again.

Now and then the finer side of his nature emerges, but this we neither force nor suppress. For a time he was aware of astral beings, and, unlike me, he was able to see 'Carl Gustav' during a trance. He is often present while we are maintaining our mediumistic contacts, and for him all this is just an everyday affair. Sometimes he even carries on trance conversations of his own with Jung (through Mira), although it must be admitted that his childlike needs became an unwelcome hindrance to our trance work. We just had to take some breaks. When he was old enough we started to conduct seminars, and Mira began promoting her special concern — the pregnancy workshops for mothers-to-be.

Manu was often glad to be allowed to greet those taking part, but then he would become bored and go back to his toys. He was always glad to sign his books with a scribble.

Mira had an interesting experience with him when he was having his bath one day. Looking into the mirror he suddenly asked whether he really looked like that. When Mira said, yes, he did, he said he thought he had black wavy hair. That was in fact how Mira had perceived him before he was born, and it was obvious that he was still seeing this image of himself.

When he was four, he went to the local kindergarten, and at six, we enrolled him in primary school, which he enjoyed very much. Now he is in the first year, and he tells us daily about the new writing skills he is learning. Recently he came up against his religious knowledge teacher. He reported with amusement that she had said that "we only live once", and when he stubbornly insisted that he knew better, the old lady gave up! "Manu, you had better believe what you believe, and I will believe my way."

All in all, he is an unusually sensitive person. On the one hand he takes it as a matter of course that he should feel equal to adults, and also he wants to be just a normal child. Up until now we have not been able to offer him the piano tuition which he was so keen on, but the prospects for this are improving. Materially we are better off today, though not, as people often assume, as a result of our books, but rather with the help of discerning sponsors who have recognised the nature and quality of our work. We feel immensely grateful for this ongoing support.

We have been quite successful in keeping the Press away from him, but we have had to go through a great deal to do so. At first we welcomed every mention in the Press, but soon it became too much. Manu remained largely untouched by this. As was to be expected, only a minority of Press reports were sympathetic. Many ranged from cutting to sarcastic. One cannot expect much else from hard-headed journalists! One example was the 'profile' in the Austrian *Spiegel*, in which the journalist used one quotation from the book, obviously intended to underline in a single sentence the banality of the alleged messages. The only message this magazine found significant was *"Now I am lying crookedly in Mummy's tummy"*. Nowadays we seldom have anything to do with the popular Press, though we no longer mind so much if they tear us to pieces.

From the many letters we have received, and from the literature we have read, it appears that the early part of the pre-natal experience we had has happened to several dozen other sensitive mothers. However, extended two-way communication with an unborn child over a longer period, such as we had, seems to be unique. Furthermore, it appears that the consciousness-enhancing process induced in parents has already saved the lives of a number of babies in the womb.

Although we certainly are not the ideal parents some readers take us to be, Manuel did make a significant confession to us a few days before I wrote this. He said quite casually that he had chosen us as parents, and he "would do the same again in his next life". I believe that if we, as parents, once again had the good fortune to be allowed the wonderful experience of a human coming into existence through us, we would let it all happen once again just as before. And we would take upon ourselves the responsibility of doing our best to inform our fellow humans of what we had experienced.

We thank you for being with us on this journey!

Notes

1. Strictly speaking, this is my fifth pregnancy. First I had a stillborn baby, then a fifth-month miscarriage (called Bernd, weighing 700g), then came David prematurely in the sixth month (lived an hour, weighed 1.05kg), then another miscarriage — *Mira*.
2. In spite of extensive researches, we have not so far heard of any similar case. The only place where we could find a parallel was in the Indian mythology of the Rig Veda — there the god Indra, as yet unborn, has a long dispute with his goddess mother about the circumstances which are to be expected at birth.
3. A loud noise in the flat below which disturbed Mira and brought her out of her meditation, caused the first message to end here.
4. To our astonishment, our baby fulfilled our request and completed the last interrupted sentence of the previous message before continuing its communication!
5. I saw him comparatively tall and slim, with dark hair and a handsome noble face, with unmistakably manly features, but also very fine, soft lines.
6. See *Dreams and Visions* earlier in the book.
7. *Mira writes*: This pure and loving guardian being likes to be near me. When I call her, it is like a fragrance — the 'breath of personality' — which accompanies me. If I concentrate on it, I can actually sense it.
8. Manuel also was not able to regard our miserable accommodation, for which we paid a high rent, as a proper home.
9. During meditation a very clear picture of him came up. I cannot explain why, but I was deeply certain that that was what he looked like: a soft, rounded forehead, large, round and wide-awake eyes and a sweet little mouth. I described him symbolically to René as a mixture between a deer and a fox! — *Mira*.
10. During communication with our baby, we often played an endless

cassette of Johann Pachelbel's Canon in D Major.

11. Heinz, our landlord's son, had visited and talked about his stepfa-
ther's behaviour.

12. A Hatha Yoga exercise.

13. While we were in the flat, earning our living together by making
Japanese futons (fleecy woollen mattresses), Mira suddenly cried out.
It was a painful but happy cry. Although it hurt, she was very pleased
about it — *René*.

14. Before Mira began her meditation, I used to put a piece of paper with
a number of questions in her hand, which seemed to me to be
important at the time — *René*.

16. This message erupted spontaneously, while we were making futon
mattresses on our living room floor. In the midst of her meditative
sewing, Mira blurted straight out what the baby was saying. I
scrambled for pen and paper. The baby realised that we were missing
some of the communication, and began again at the first sentence, so
that nothing was lost!

17. We treated ourselves to a feast for five people in the Indian restaurant
'Shakuntla'.

18. I had been invited to Majorca for a sort of therapy holiday — in
Austria, spiritual healing is still forbidden! During this time I used to
dance calmly in the street, my mind filled with the thought of having
a baby. My 'patient' said I should get the idea out of my head, since I
did not have the resources to feed a child anyway. But with my last
coins I rang René at home to tell him I was now absolutely certain I
wanted a baby.

19. Alfred, our natural-food grocer, came to visit us with his lively kids
in tow.

20. I had been rubbing herb oil into Mira's now very rounded tummy
and concentrating entirely on the baby as I did so — *René*.

22. After a long discussion, we decided not to publish the name given
here by the baby.

23. *Embryo*, from Greek, means bud, seedling, fruit of the body. In
medicine, the embryo is renamed a *foetus* (from Latin) from the third
month onwards. Our baby does not keep to this terminology, but
calls itself an embryo right up to birth.

24. A rather demanding 'friend' would simply not desist or go away.

25. This is the imaginal scenery of a more subtle sphere of being.

26. At this time we were in the process of moving from Linz to Pension
Waldesruh, in the country. The apartment was so dilapidated that the

town council had put a demolition order on it.

27. Possibly Manuji is referring to 'astral' dwelling places.

28. The industrial air of Linz was one of the reasons we moved to the country. The contamination attacked Mira's eyes and lungs, and even the birch trees in a neighbour's garden.

29. It was the LP of George Winston playing a piano version of the Canon in D Major by Pachelbel.

30. My brother's three-year old son had of his own accord given the baby his own rattle, Manuji's first toy — *René*.

31. René had rung up his mother and asked whether it would be possible to have a little financial support toward our setting up a new home. Since his father absolutely refused any such help, my husband spoke angrily. This was what Manuji was picking up on — *Mira*.

32. I used to pack the futons we made into great rolls and dragged them through the hallway and out of the flat. It was tiring doing it. Mira was unable to help me any longer, so I was always rather exhausted afterwards.

33. Often in my mind I put a protective covering around me and the baby, in order to protect us from dissonant vibrations — *Mira*.

34. A t.v.

35. I let healing energy flow through my tummy to the baby — *Mira*.

36. We lay snuggled up together for hours (the heating often didn't work), and motionlessly loved each other *Mira*.

37. During meditation.

38. Mostly I meditate in the half-lotus position, or kneeling Japanese-style.

39. I used to wind a shawl around me to protect the baby from noise — *Mira*.

40. A little girl of six in the family downstairs has been suffering from a longterm psychosomatic cough.

41. I had bought the Winston music because Manuji had said how much he wanted to play the piano — *René*.

42. We had a row with the landlord over urgent repairs he was not doing, and this disturbed me — *Mira*.

43. From the other apartments.

44. I called René in Vienna, where he was working. He urged me to ask Lydia for a refuge. She picked me up shortly after from this madhouse. The second voice belonged to a friend of Lydia's.

45. Lydia's deep voice.

46. Half-a-dozen of Lydia's friends visited. It was an amusing interlude.

47. I used to take a lot of long walks in the woods, in order to escape from Pension Waldesruh, and to enjoy the true woodland peace. Since there were no woods close to Lydia's, this stopped — *Mira.*

48. Mira used to lovingly look after our flowers. She would talk to them and irradiate them with her hands. She was particularly fond of a little Spanish chestnut sapling of the same age as Manuji — *René.*

49. The whole afternoon I had been talking to Lydia about her case of infantile paralysis, about the mental effects, the possible causes and about my opinion that all diseases can be cured.

50. As all other rooms at Lydia's were through-rooms, she was extra kind to let us use her bedroom.

51. A farmhouse was advertised in a newspaper, which I went to view, but like a lot of others, it was a let-down.

52. It seems that Manuji already had a sense that something was about to happen to us.

53. Noises were caused by the pain recorder, the infusion apparatus and various metallic medical instruments.

54. The voices of nurses and doctors.

55. I prayed. Then I felt the presence of my spirit-friends as a very dear, strong, warm and helpful vibration. Sometimes I saw that someone was there with my inner eye.

56. The effect of the glucose in the infusion was beginning.

57. In the ward next to me, a baby was born by caesarean section. This baby's cries shook me very deeply and made me sad. I couldn't help crying for it. I didn't know at the time about the caesarean — the midwife told me about it later.

58. A few times each day, the babies, about six of them, would be wheeled down the corridor to the individual 'sick rooms'. We could hear them crying through the door of our room.

59. Various medicines had an effect on the amniotic fluid. Later, I had eaten some bread with sugar-free jam on it, and that seems to have sweetened the amniotic fluids.

60. Before the messages began again, we had had a difference of opinion about whether or not to carry on with the book. René wanted me by all means to establish contact again. I felt I was still too weak, but then I did it all the same, for my husband's sake.

61. From the window in the room I could see what the birds were doing in a neighbouring large tree.

62. This is caused by the medication I was receiving.

63. I had asked Mira to try communicating with the baby in both

mornings and evenings, since there was perhaps only a little time left for doing so — *René*.

64. René had made a copy of the messages to date, which he had laid on the table by my bed. I kept reading it and pondering over each part — *Mira*.

65. We had been arguing over something — it must have been insignificant, because neither of us can remember what it was!

66. When I was to have my ultrasound examination, I was wheeled down to the basement. We had talked to the junior doctor about finding out the sex of the baby. He thought it was 'possibly a girl' — the position of the baby's body prevented being sure — *Mira*.

67. This refers to my playing the alpha-wave music through headphones to relax me. Sometimes I held the headphones over my stomach — *Mira*.

68. I experienced a vivid daydream.

69. I touched Mira's stomach gently with my hand and spoke directly to Manuji from as close a distance as possible. I told him that I thought what he was doing was really wonderful and that it made me well able to adjust myself to fatherhood, plus other things — *René*.

70. Here, Emanuel was recognising himself as Manuji for the first time, since, after discovering the meaning of the name, I had lovingly called him by it several times — *Mira*.

71. In an attack of doubt, I lost courage, and the feeling that all would go well — *Mira*.

72. This refers to a dream I had about 4 months previously — see the chapter 'Dreams and Visions' — *Mira*.

73. This seems to have something to do with the medicines I had taken — *Mira*.

74. The same picture as I saw during the very first message — *Mira*.

75. In spite of my request not to be disturbed between seven and nine in the evening, a particularly inquisitive nurse suddenly entered the room. That irritated me so much that I was not able to concentrate fully on the message that evening. René, who usually would sit by the door to prevent disturbance, was not there that evening — *Mira*.

76. On the second ultrasound examination, the doctor was able to see the baby's sex clearly, and show it to us on the screen.

77. I was sleeping 25km away at my parents' house — *René*.

78. As a father, I count this as one of the most wonderful experiences of this exciting time. I was in an office in Linz, using an electric typewriter. I was typing out a fair copy of the messages to show a

publisher. While I was typing away there for nights on end, I remembered that our son had, early on, said he would give a report about 'heaven'. I had a burning interest in this, and needed to make it clear to my son. I rang Mira at the clinic, and asked her to hold the telephone receiver to her tummy. I explained my interest to Manuji and added some further questions. I gave him a choice of subjects I would like him to discuss. His reaction was amazing, and made us very happy — *René*.

79. This refers to the ultrasound scan.

80. This was the doctor, who was kind and sympathetic as he did the ultrasound scan.

81. The new-born babies were on the fourth floor of the clinic. On the third floor were the labour wards and rooms, and on the second floor were large and small rooms for patients. Manuji was on his way from the second to the fourth floor.

82. A few days later we discovered there was a special incubator on the fourth floor, but we weren't able to find out whether there had been a little girl in it. We did not have access to this section, and also didn't want to reveal the reasons for our curiosity.

83. Mira rang me up in the office in Linz immediately after she had finished writing down this message. She phoned the text through and, completely euphoric, I immediately typed it out — *René*.

84. Financial support.

85. These are micro-organisms which live in the amniotic fluid. A doctor informed us that these are presumably 'Endobionts', which can be seen moving around and glimmering under a dark-field microscope.

86. Before this contact, René had placed his hands on my now very large stomach and asked Manuji to tell us something about abortion. The newspapers at that time were preoccupied with this matter again, and people were demonstrating for and against it in the streets as well — *Mira*.

87. During the previous few days, we parents had been having little differences of opinion on account of this book. I had rung up various authorities in pre-natal psychology and informed them about what had been happening. I wanted to give 'experts' an opportunity to give objective assessments of our experiences. I thought that this would be necessary if we were to be believed later. Understandably, Mira wanted to be left in peace, and had no wish to saddle herself with anything like that. However, she finally agreed to my plan. But then the specialists took very little interest in us — which is difficult

for me to understand to this day. *René.*

88. His birth was now finally really at hand. After I had devoted all my energy to making this communication between my son and his mother possible in the circumstances which prevailed, I was unwilling to accept that the messages should just end abruptly. So I kept on asking Mira to try to re-establish contact. However, with the best will in the world, she was unable to write any more, because the labour pains were already too severe. I then suggested that she should try to make contact all the same and simply say out loud what she was hearing inwardly. I could then write it all down. Amazingly, this was successful — *René.*